Testimonials

I was diagnosed in 2010 with stage 4b lung cancer in my upper lobe of my left lung. I underwent 35 radiation treatments and 6 chemotherapy infusions. The tumor is inoperable but is in remission. I am now a five-year survivor and feel great, with my next check-up scheduled for the end of March 2016.

In order to change some of my dietary habits, I contacted Mary McAlary. I knew of the health problems that she had endured and how changing her diet had improved her overall health. I have changed my diet and have noticed how much better I do feel; when I do have something that I should not consume, my body lets me know about it with stomach cramps and just not feeling well.

I still stay in contact with Mary just in case I need her advice. Mary is a wonderful coach to have in my corner!

Sincerely, E.F.

I was diagnosed in the winter of 2013–2014 with stage 3 squamous non-small cell lung cancer. The tumor is located in the bronchial tube in the upper lobe of my right lung. It is inoperable but treatable. After going through 35 radiation sessions and 15 chemotherapy treatments and hearing from nutritionists at the hospital, the decision was made to seek out the advice of Mary McAlary. I had known of Mary's condition and how her diet change had made huge improvements in her well-being. So I decided to give it a shot—nothing ventured, nothing gained.

To be honest, the changes were difficult at first. But after meeting with Mary periodically, and with her continued support, I could really feel a difference in my activity level and with other aspects of my life. My blood sugar level has been maintained, and my cholesterol level has been under 200 for quite a while. All of my blood work levels have been normal for the last 10 months of 2015. If I do stray off of my diet, my system lets me know about it within a very short time.

I cannot thank Mary for enough for all of her help and inspiration through the changes that have been made in my diet and well-being.

Thank you Mary!!

Sincerely, B.F.

Friends, family and my doctors tell me that I look great. My energy level is so much better! I have been able to stop taking pain medicine, and for the first time in over thirteen years, I am no longer taking prednisone.

I am enjoying eating healthier foods and feeling great. All thanks to Mary.

P.L.

Years ago my mother was diagnosed with MS. After a long battle with doctors, medications, and pain, she knew she needed a new path and some new ideas, which lead her to study nutrition. I had my hesitations and was afraid to see her stray away from her well-trained specialists and what they were telling her to do and instead go natural and holistic. But she was brave, put one foot in front of the other, and embarked on a life-changing journey that not only affected her, but also made everyone around her healthier and "food aware" too! The transformation and story is remarkable. I watched her improve every day as a result of her diet.

Back when this new lifestyle started, I never believed that food, nutrition, and diet could affect someone in such a powerful and healing way. I knew healthy foods were good for you and bad foods were not, but I never understood or believed that if you learn how to eat for your own body and for your ailments, food can actually heal you. I learned from my mother to think of my body like a machine—if you fuel it with the best possible options, it will run beautifully. Learning to control what you put in your body is the most valuable information that there is and a movement all should take part in.

So thank you to this incredible author I am lucky enough to call my mother—for being brave, for learning so much about healing yourself, for teaching and helping others, and for showing me how to be healthy and care for myself the way nature intended. And of course, thank you for sharing some of your delicious recipes in this book!

Marisa Morello

GO GREEN
FOR WELLNESS
Smoothies, Juices, Green Recipes

Practical Advice for
Achieving Good Health

MARY McALARY
Author of *The Fighting Spirit*

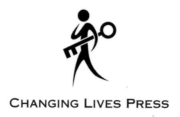

CHANGING LIVES PRESS

Disclaimer: Please consult your physician before beginning this or any other dietary changes, especially if you are currently taking any prescription or over-the-counter medications, are pregnant, are a minor, or have any type of medical condition.

The information contained in this book is designed to maintain good health and does not claim to treat or cure disease. It is not a substitute for regular medical care.

Always consult your physician for medical advice before beginning any dietary program.

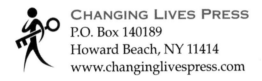

CHANGING LIVES PRESS
P.O. Box 140189
Howard Beach, NY 11414
www.changinglivespress.com

Library of Congress Cataloging-in-Publication Data is available through the Library of Congress.

ISBN-13: 978-0-99094-243-6

Editor: Lisa Espinoza
Cover and Interior design: Gary A. Rosenberg

Printed in the United States of America

10   9   8   7   6   5   4   3   2   1

Contents

Acknowledgments

Throughout my adult life, being a mother has been my greatest blessing. I vowed to take good care of myself so that I could raise my children to become happy, responsible adults. I am pleased to say that my children, now grown, are amazing people who are caring, intelligent, and successful. As my grandchildren came along, I committed to being healthy and to participate in their lives and the lives of future grandchildren. I want to see them grow up and experience all of the joys life has to offer.

Prior to my diagnosis with MS, I was an active, vibrant grandmother who enjoyed playing with the next generation of her matriarchy. MS began to rob me of that pleasure. I was unable to pick up my grandchildren or to play with them anymore. The pain of not being able to be the person I used to be inspired me to do all that I could to heal and be the Grammy I wanted to be. Today I am in remission and plan to remain that way.

I dedicate this book to my grandchildren. To Kasey, who will begin college in the fall of 2016, who is a leader and doesn't go with the flow. Stay strong in your individuality and character. To Jake, who has the kindest soul and makes everyone feel so very special. If everyone in the world had your heart, it would be a beautiful place. I cherish our times together playing pool. Thanks for letting me win now and then. To Ryan, my free-spirited, unique, talented granddaughter who rocks and has a keen understanding of the world. You make me feel adored. To Tucker, my fearless boy whose smiles brighten the world and whose hugs capture my heart. To my grandchildren yet to be born, for keeping me inspired to continue fighting for my health. Hopefully I will live to be 110 so that I can enjoy the abundant happiness and love so generously bestowed upon me.

Foreword

My first book, *The Fighting Spirit,* is the story of my battle against multiple sclerosis. Today my diagnosis has been changed to "benign" MS. I am grateful to say that I am healthy and medication free. My mission is to pay forward the blessings that I have received by sharing the knowledge that helped transform my health—and my life.

When asked to write this second book, *Go Green for Wellness,* I decided to include a continuation of my story, including the most important health habits that have contributed to my well-being. Perhaps the greatest positive impact on my health came as a result of my choice to go green—to make fruits and vegetables (not just the green ones) the centerpiece of my diet. I found that juices and smoothies were a simple, delicious way to consume more produce than I might if I were to eat them on a plate. So I am including some of my favorite smoothie and juice recipes. I also really enjoy eating my greens, therefore, I have also included some great green recipes for you to enjoy on your plate as well.

Since I began my journey to health in 2007, I have learned something new each and every day. *Go Green for Wellness* is a compilation of over eight years of research information that I have discovered during my recovery. I hope that it will inspire and educate others to make important changes that will result in healthier, richer lives.

Whatever your "fight" may be, whether it is a health crisis, a personal battle, or just a desire to be healthier, my prayer is that this book will truly make a positive difference in your life.

CHAPTER 1

My Biggest Challenge

In June of 2004, I faced the biggest challenge of my life—the initial physical attack of an illness that would ultimately be identified as multiple sclerosis. I was told that MS is incurable and that I should prepare myself for life in a wheelchair. I began the prescribed medications and became very ill. I felt alone and frightened, and I was in constant pain. I could see the concern and fear in the eyes of my family and friends who were witnessing my decline in health. After several months, I decided to discontinue the medication injections that were prescribed.

The ensuing three years were a nightmare of continuing pain and disabilities. I suffered from severe neuropathy, trigeminal neuralgia, restless leg syndrome, spasms, numbness, and side effects of the medications that I was taking in an attempt to relieve my ailments. I was falling, foot dragging, and at times needed a cane to walk. In 2007, I was taking 18 prescription medications per day to help me function.

I finally reached my limit and decided to find a healthier approach to managing my disease. I attended the Institute for Integrative Nutrition and began to change my diet and my life. By April of 2008, I was medication free, and in June of 2008, I received my certification as a Holistic Health Coach.

Over the years since my diagnosis and subsequent healing, I have become aware of countless individuals who are suffering from the often-debilitating disease of MS. I have been asked frequently just how I achieved wellness. What did you eat? What did you do to overcome such a serious health challenge? This book is my response to those questions.

My challenge today is to keep acquiring knowledge, to maintain my health, and to continue sharing what I learn to help others.

CHAPTER 2

The Good Ole Days When Food Was Food

It was a simpler life when I was young. We didn't have a television until I was six years old. There were no computers, Internet, or social networking sites. There were no nuclear power plants or trash incinerators in our area, nor were potentially toxic plastics used as extensively as they are today. There was far less in our environment to worry about.

I believe our food supply was much healthier than it is today. We bought locally from nearby farms and grew our produce in our own gardens. We had little access to fruits and vegetables from areas outside of New England, especially after the harvest months. Canning was a 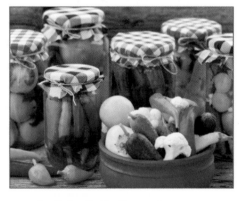 family affair every fall so that we had fresh fruits and vegetables throughout the winter. Fertilizer was not synthetic but merely cow manure from the farm across the street. The butchers were local, and we purchased our groceries from small family-owned grocery stores. Chain stores like WalMart, Stop & Shop, BJ's, and Costco were still decades away.

My grandparents lived a few houses down the street from my family's home. My grandfather raised chickens in a coop in the backyard of their house. As a child, I used to gather eggs for the family. My grandfather would eat the chickens—much to my dismay, because I had named them all.

I grew up across the street from several farms. My brothers and I would help our neighbors milk their cows. Our reward was to drink the raw milk and skim the cream from the tops of the buckets to whip or churn into fresh butter. Glass-bottled milk was delivered to us by a milkman from a local farm.

Those were the days my friends. . . .

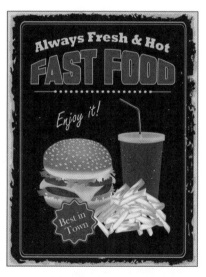

In my early teens, the fast-food revolution came into existence. The first fast-food hamburger restaurant opened in the area, and we were quite excited to purchase 15-cent hamburgers. It was a new experience. We would ride to Howdy Beefburger or Adventure Car Hop and get a hamburger, fries, and a shake for less than 50 cents. We never considered the ingredients of those foods or where they came from. We simply trusted the sources.

Farms began disappearing, and mini-mansions began to pop up. Modern farming techniques were beginning to dramatically change the quality of what we ate. Cattle and livestock were being injected with hormones to promote fast growth and antibiotics to prevent disease as they were being raised in large warehouses. They were no longer fed the grains and grasses of the free range.

Along came supermarkets, and the mom-and-pop grocery

stores began to disappear as well. The time-saving convenience of shopping for everything you needed in one place was quite appealing. Produce from other countries was abundant in the winter months. However, because of the distance and time to travel to the stores, preservatives were used to get the food from the farm to the supermarket. We never thought about nutrition and the effects of chemicals and additives in our foods because we were accustomed to eating local, fresh food.

Products began to have a long shelf life. Chemical sweeteners, synthetic preservatives, and additives became common ingredients and enabled busy people to enjoy frozen dinners and processed foods that required little time to prepare. To most, it seemed that this was an improvement, but eventually the ill effects of fast food began to manifest themselves.

Now decades later, our addiction to sugar and processed fast foods is evident. According to the National Institutes of Health, more than two-thirds (68.8 percent) of adults are considered to be overweight or obese. More than 1 in 20 (6.3 percent) are considered to be extremely obese. Obesity puts an individual at risk for a variety of ailments including diabetes, hypertension, cardiovascular disease, stroke, pulmonary disease, reproductive disorders, osteoarthritis, and cancer, among others.

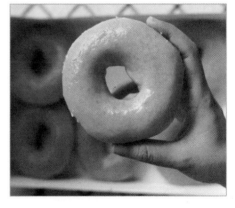

The United States Department of Health and Services reports that 14.7 to 23.5 million people in this country are affected by autoimmune diseases. These diseases often cause debilitating symptoms and result in enormous medical expenses, loss of productivity and ability to work. Because these diseases are one of the leading causes of death for young and middle aged women, they impose an exceptional burden on families and on society.

In most cases, when a disease is diagnosed, patients are prescribed medications, many times without any discussion of

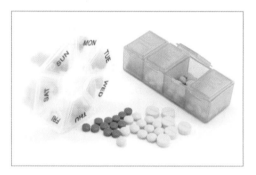

possible lifestyle changes that could create a more positive outlook with regard to their health. Those medications then produce adverse side effects that are often, in turn, treated with even more medications. Just count the number of people you know who have to use those plastic pillboxes to organize their multiple daily medications. I was certainly headed in that direction.

Even though I have always loved to cook and made my meals mostly from scratch, I wasn't choosing the healthiest ingredients for my homemade meals. When a health crisis forced me to re-examine my diet, I was able to successfully change course and will continue to do everything in my power to keep it that way.

One of the changes I made was to be very aware of everything I put in my grocery cart. In the past, I rarely paid attention to labels, but now I read every label, and if it has ingredients that I cannot pronounce or do not recognize, I put it back on the shelf.

I used to blindly accept the food industry's standards and products. No more. For example, I was unaware of the importance of high-fiber, low-sugar foods until I attended the Institute for Integrative Nutrition. Since that time, I have made great strides to live a "clean" life by focusing on organic foods and products that are high in fiber, low in sugar.

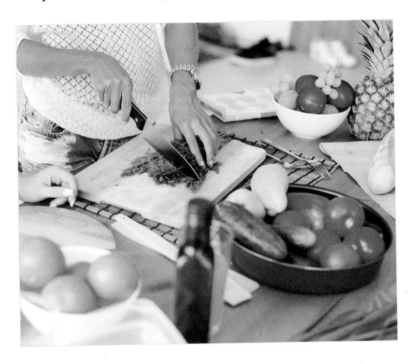

When I first started down this road to rediscovering good health, it was like learning a new language. Discovering new methods of cooking and revising my stale vocabulary of ingredients was exciting. Quinoa, turmeric, kohlrabi, and coconut oil opened up a whole new world of flavor for me. My food vocabulary has grown tremendously!

Since those early days, I have prepared recipes from a vast array of dietary theories such as raw food, vegan, vegetarian, gluten free, paleo, and macrobiotic, among others. Each recipe is prepared consciously—choosing every ingredient with an eye for its ability to positively or negatively affect the health of those on the other end of the fork.

My years of research have led to countless "aha" moments about what I put in and on my body. For the sake of simplicity, I can condense them to a few words of advice: read every label; choose healthy, whole foods; and buy organic whenever possible. We will talk more about that in the next chapter. These choices have made a tremendous positive impact on my health. This process didn't happen overnight, and it is an ongoing journey. Every day I learn something new and continue to work toward making positive changes.

CHAPTER 3

Organic
Is the Best Choice

"Organic" has become a popular buzzword in recent years. But organic is more than just the latest fad. In this chapter, we will talk about how choosing an organic diet leads to optimal health for us and for our planet. I have done extensive research on this topic, and one of the most concise treatments I've discovered is by Renee Loux in a 2011 online article in *Prevention*. Much of the information in this chapter is adapted from that article.

Organic farming supports a healthy planet. By utilizing sustainable techniques, including crop rotation and chemical abstinence, fertile soil is maintained. Farming in harmony with nature allows each element of the ecosystem to play its unique role, thereby ensuring a sustainable future for our children.

Non-organic farming does not honor the harmony of nature. Pesticides used in conventional farming adversely impact wildlife, insects, frogs, birds, and soil, compromising their ability to fulfill their part in maintaining a healthy ecosystem. In addition, agricultural chemicals, pesticides, and fertilizers are contaminating our environment and poisoning our water supplies.

Most conventional food is hybridized for larger, more attractive food products, thereby decreasing the variety of crops being grown. In fact, in the last century, there has been a 75 percent decrease in crop diversity. Why is this a problem? Growing diverse crops is critical to survival. One example lies in the great potato famine in Ireland—an entire crop consisting of only a few varieties of potatoes was killed, and millions of people died of starvation. Today only a handful of varieties of potatoes dominate the marketplace, whereas thousands of varieties were once available. Compare this to the environmentally sound method of growing indigenous strains that are tolerant of regional conditions such as droughts and pests.

While we may wholeheartedly disagree with current nonorganic farming practices, our tax dollars are at work subsidizing billions of dollars for a farm bill that heavily favors the commercial farming industry. A study at Cornell University determined that the cost of a head of commercial iceberg lettuce, typically purchased at 49 cents a head, actually costs more than $3 dollars a head when hidden costs are considered. The study factored in the costs of federal subsidies, pesticide regulation and testing, and hazardous waste cleanup.

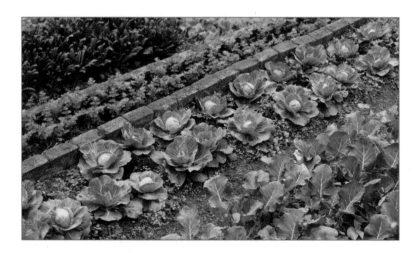

We need to let our voices be heard by choosing not to support unhealthy policies and practices that drive our trillion-dollar food industry. Cast your vote for a sustainable future for generations to come by spending your dollars in the organic sector.

While eating organically supports our planet's health, probably the most powerful motivator to go green is the personal health benefit that accompanies an organic lifestyle. When you eat foods that are free of chemicals and full of nutritious, robust flavor, you are choosing to give your body exactly what it needs to thrive.

Organic foods have more nutrients, vitamins, minerals, enzymes, and micronutrients than commercially grown foods due to soil management and sustainable practices by responsible standards. According to *The Journal of Alternative and Complementary Medicine,* five servings of organically grown vegetables (such as lettuce, spinach, carrots, potatoes, and cabbage) provide an adequate allowance of vitamin C, whereas the same number of servings of conventionally grown vegetables does not. In addition to all of these nutritional benefits, organic foods taste better because nourished, well-balanced soil produces healthy, strong plants. This is especially true with heirloom varieties, which are cultivated for taste over appearance.

On the flip side, let's look at what our bodies take in when we fill them with non-organic foods. At present, more than 600 active chemicals are registered for agricultural use in America. Every year, the average chemical pesticide application equals about 16 pounds per person. The National Academy of Sciences reports that 90 percent of the chemicals applied to foods have not been tested for long-term health effects before being deemed "safe." The most dangerous and toxic pesticides require special testing methods, which are rarely, if ever, employed by the FDA.

The Food Revolution Network (www.foodrevolution.org) details a compelling list of reasons to avoid pesticides. Various studies have linked the use of pesticides to asthma, allergies,

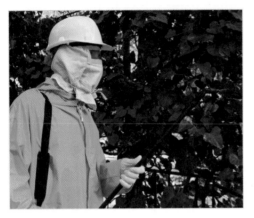 weight gain and obesity, birth defects, infertility, cancer, Alzheimer's disease, diabetes, autism, Parkinson's disease, and damage to the liver and kidneys. It makes good sense to eat organic since certified organic standards prohibit the use of harmful pesticides.

The Environmental Protection Agency (EPA) reports that a majority of pesticide intake comes from meal, poultry, fish, eggs, and dairy products because these foods are high on the food chain. For instance, a large fish that eats a smaller fish that eats even smaller fish accumulates all of the toxins of the chain, especially in the fatty tissue. Cows, chickens, and pigs are fed animal parts, by-products, fishmeal, and grains that are laden with toxins and chemicals. In fact, more than 90 percent of the pesticides Americans consume are found in the fat and tissue of meat and dairy products.

In addition, tens of millions of pounds of antibiotics are used in animal feed every year. Many scientists and experts warn that rampant use of antibiotics in animal feed, like penicillin and tetracycline, will breed an epidemic that medicine has no defense against. Karim Ahmed, PhD, a senior scientist at the Natural Resources Defense Council (NRDC) states that it "is perhaps one of the most serious public health problems the country faces. We're talking about rendering many of the most important antibiotics ineffective."

Farmers in the U.S. have been giving sex hormones and growth hormones to cattle to artificially increase the amount of meat and milk the cattle produce without requiring extra feed. The hormones fed to cows cannot be broken down, even at high temperatures, so they remain in complete form and pass directly to the consumer's diet when the meat is eaten.

This information should not be taken lightly. rBGH or rBST, the growth hormones in milk, are genetically modified and have been directly linked to cancer, especially in women. Besides cancer, consumption of growth hormones in our food supply has been implicated in other major concerns for Americans including early onset of puberty, growth of tumors, and genetic problems. While the jury is still out on the issue here in America, Europe's scientific community agrees that there is no acceptably safe level for daily intake of any of the hormones currently used in the United States and has subsequently banned all growth hormones.

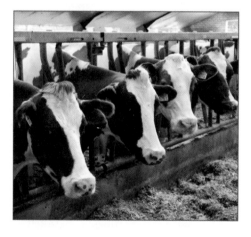

Choosing products free of hormones is of the utmost importance, especially for children, pregnant women, and nursing mothers. The only way to avoid consuming these harmful additives is to choose an organic diet.

Chemicals, growth hormones, antibiotics, and pesticides aren't the only dangerous elements to avoid. Genetically engineered (GE) food and genetically modified organisms (GMOs) are contaminating our food supply at an alarming rate, with repercussions beyond our current understanding. Because organically grown food cannot be genetically modified in any way, choosing organic is the only way to be sure that foods that have been genetically engineered stay out of your diet.

GMOs are living organisms whose genetic material has been artificially manipulated in a laboratory through genetic engineering, or GE. According to the Non-GMO Project, this relatively new science creates unstable combinations of plant, animal, bacteria, and viral genes that do not occur in nature or through traditional crossbreeding methods.

Virtually all commercial GMOs are engineered to allow pesticide application while leaving the marketable food product intact. Despite promises by the biotech industry, genetically modified foods do not offer increased yield, drought tolerance, enhanced nutrition, or any other consumer benefit. At the same time, there is mounting evidence that GMOs and the industry that promotes their use can be linked to environmental damage, violation of farmers' and consumers' rights, and health problems.

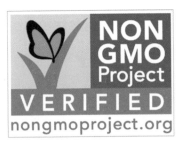

Most developed nations do not consider GMOs to be safe for consumption. In more than 60 countries around the world, including Australia, Japan, and all of the countries in the European Union, there are significant restrictions or outright bans on the production and sale of GMOs. In the U.S., the government has approved GMOs based on studies conducted by the same corporations that created them and profit from their sale.

Why contribute to the GMO industry while also experimenting with your own health? When choosing foods for yourself and your family, look for the Non-GMO Project butterfly sticker that is displayed on non-GMO foods.

CHAPTER 4

Choose Your Produce Wisely

While it is always safest to eat organic, there may be times when you have limited or no availability of organic produce. The following lists will help you make wise choices in these situations. The Environmental Working Group (EWG), in association with Dr. Andrew Weil, compiled these lists of the most contaminated and least contaminated produce. This information, published in 2014, is based on nine years of pesticide testing results and takes into account the typical method of washing and preparation for each type of produce. The foods on the first list, the "Dirty Dozen," should only be consumed if you are able to find them organically grown.

The following list, the "Clean 15," includes conventionally grown fruits and vegetables that tested lowest for pesticides.

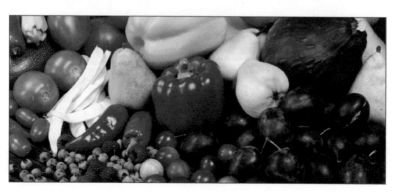

THE "DIRTY DOZEN"
FOODS YOU SHOULD ALWAYS BUY ORGANIC

1. Apples
2. Strawberries
3. Grapes
4. Celery
5. Peaches
6. Spinach

7. Sweet bell peppers
8. Nectarines (imported)
9. Cucumbers
10. Cherry tomatoes
11. Snap peas (imported)
12. Potatoes

In addition, avoid non-organic hot peppers and blueberries (domestic) as they may contain organophosphate insecticides, which EWG characterizes as "highly toxic" and of special concern.

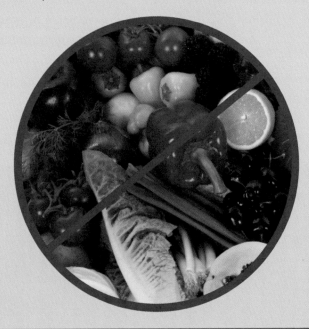

THE "CLEAN 15"
FOODS YOU DON'T HAVE TO BUY ORGANIC

1. Avocados
2. Sweet corn
3. Pineapples
4. Cabbage
5. Sweet peas (frozen)
6. Onions
7. Asparagus
8. Mangoes
9. Papayas
10. Kiwi
11. Eggplant
12. Grapefruit
13. Cantaloupe (domestic)
14. Cauliflower
15. Sweet potatoes

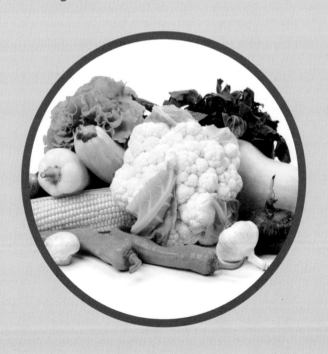

CHAPTER 5

Your Mother Was Right— Eat Your Veggies

Only about one-quarter of American adults eat three or more servings of vegetables a day. If you are not getting enough greens in your diet, you are missing out on one of the most potent prescriptions for optimal health. And for those of us who are parents, we have the challenging responsibility to ensure that our children are eating enough vegetables. We can carry out our secret mission by hiding vegetables in recipes, juices, and smoothies.

If possible, purchase your greens within a day or two before you intend to use them. Make sure that the leaves are firm and are not discolored or wilted. Wash and dry them well. If you are not going to use them immediately, store them in your refrigerator. Remember, the fresher, the better, and buy organic whenever possible to avoid pesticides.

Greens are loaded with magnesium, iron, potassium, phosphorous, zinc, and vitamins A, C, E, and K. They are also a good source of calcium, which is especially helpful for those who choose not to consume dairy products. They are chock full of fiber, folic acid, chlorophyll, and antioxidants as well as many other micronutrients and phytochemicals that can reduce inflammation, eliminate carcinogens, rid the body of old cells, and maintain DNA.

Dark leafy greens improve circulation, purify the blood, strengthen the immune system, and promote healthy intestinal flora. They improve liver, gall bladder, and kidney function and clear congestion by reducing the production of mucus.

Adding vegetables to your diet lowers the risk of certain types of cancer, stroke, high blood pressure, type 2 diabetes, heart disease, Alzheimer's disease and digestive disorders, just to name a few.

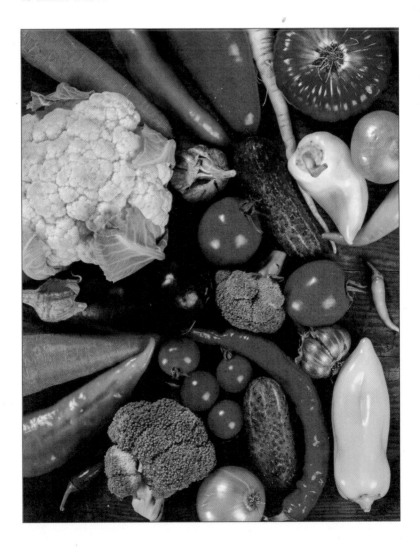

Speaking of digestive health, we have heard in recent years how important it is to get enough fiber in our diets, right? When you think fiber, don't forget your greens. With between 3–6 grams of fiber in a one-cup serving, green vegetables help our bodies eliminate waste and toxins.

The anti-inflammatory properties of greens can help control blood pressure and regulate blood sugar. Chlorophyll, also found in leafy greens, supports our internal system, and studies report that it may reverse or slow down the aging process. Leafy greens improve the quality of your skin, giving you a healthy, youthful glow. Because greens are high in fiber and low in calories and carbohydrates, they are great for the digestive tract and aid in weight loss.

In the past, it was thought that fats, proteins, carbohydrates, vitamins, and minerals were all of the nutrients needed for our health. Today, we know that there is another essential group of nutrients needed for optimal health known as phytochemicals, also referred to as phytonutrients. These are often concentrated in the skins of many fruits and vegetables and are responsible for their color, scent, hue, and flavor. Foods rich in phytochemicals are tomatoes, grapes, garlic, sweet potatoes, red onions and cabbage, broccoli, kale, spinach, parsley, green tea, blueberries, raspberries, blackberries, and melons just to name a few.

Some phytonutrients help our cells communicate with each other more efficiently, help to prevent mutations at a cellular level, and are anti-inflammatory. Others are potent antioxidants that help prevent cancer, heart disease, aging, and chronic diseases by boosting the immune system.

The best-known phytonutrients are carotenoids, flavonoids, polyphenols, indoles, lignans and isoflavones. Carotenoids are the yellow, orange, and red pigment in fruits and vegetables as well as in dark green, leafy vegetables. Beta-carotene is a carotenoid. Its usual yellow color may be masked by chlorophyll, the green pigment in vegetables. Flavonoids are the red pigments found in grape skins and citrus fruits. Polyphenols are found in green tea and berries. Cruciferous vegetables such as broccoli and cauliflower contain indoles; lignans are found in flaxseed; and isoflavones are found in legumes such as peanuts, lentils, and soy. The phytochemicals, antioxidants, carotenoids and flavonoids found in greens help to protect your eyes and have been shown to prevent certain cancers.

Flavonoid and carotenoids have more health promoting properties when consumed together in the same food than separately. Organic fruits and vegetables are a great source of these important nutrients.

So why wouldn't we include these power-packed health promoters in our daily diets? Well, many of us have veggie aversion because of past experience. Bland flavor, unappealing

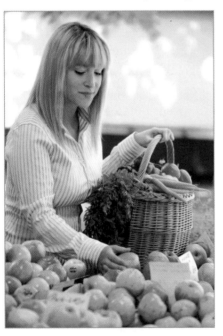

consistency, and memories of punishment for hiding them under the napkin. Or we have the preconceived notion that in order to make veggies a part of our daily diet, we will need to quit our job or ignore our family to make time for all the necessary slicing, dicing, and overall food prep. Any of these ring a bell? I'm here to tell you, veggies can be delicious and simple to prepare, and I will prove it in the recipes to come.

CHAPTER 6

Set Your Goals

What are your goals? Perhaps you are interested in having more energy, losing weight, addressing a health challenge, supporting a friend, or just living a healthier lifestyle. Many of my clients come to me wanting to achieve all of these goals, and every one of them can be achieved by committing to a healthy dietary change. You will have much more energy, burn more calories, lose weight, and feel and look great. Your example will inspire others around you to begin to set their own positive life-changing goals.

Each of us is unique. What works for one person may not work for another. The key is to listen to your body and learn what is best for you. We all have our food likes and dislikes.

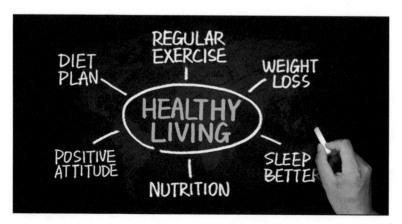

Many of us have food allergies or sensitivities that we may or may not be aware of. This is all-important information to be aware of when embarking on a food lifestyle change.

It is very helpful to keep a food diary. By doing so, you will have a written log of the foods that make you feel energized and those that do not. You will begin to understand which foods make you feel bloated, tired, or just not your best. Use the pages provided at the end of this chapter to keep a daily record of what you are eating and drinking and how you feel. Alternatively, you can purchase a notebook or use your cell phone or computer to keep your daily record. Check to see which applications are available to track your diet and progress. Make the process as simple as possible so that you will stick with it.

As you keep your diary, write what you eat for breakfast. Note how you felt several hours later. Were you hungry and tired or full of energy, focused, and alert? Do the same for snacks, lunch, and dinner.

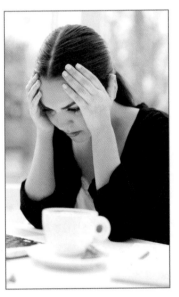

An example of the side effects you may experience has to do with your morning cup of coffee. Do you get a headache if you do not drink coffee? If you drink too much coffee, do you feel shaky and restless or experience insomnia? Do you feel a surge of energy followed by fatigue several hours later and find yourself craving another cup? This is, of course, related to the caffeine in the coffee, but other foods (and over-the-counter medications) that contain caffeine may cause similar reactions—non-herbal tea, chocolate, and soda, to name a few.

WHAT ARE YOUR GOALS?

Writing them down will help you to achieve them.

_____

_____

_____

_____

_____

_____

_____

_____

_____

_____

_____

_____

_____

_____

_____

_____

_____

_____

WHAT ARE YOUR GOALS?

Writing them down will help you to achieve them.

_____

_____

_____

_____

_____

_____

_____

_____

_____

_____

_____

_____

_____

_____

_____

_____

_____

_____

_____

_____

_____

WHAT ARE YOUR GOALS?

Writing them down will help you to achieve them.

WHAT ARE YOUR GOALS?

Writing them down will help you to achieve them.

CHAPTER 7

Stress Less

Any discussion about improving our lifestyle choices must include a few words about stress. Making choices that help us manage our stress levels is key to maintaining optimum health.

A study at Carnegie Mellon University found that chronic psychological stress is associated with a weakening of the body's ability to regulate inflammatory processes in the body. The leader of the study, Sheldon Cohen, said, "When under stress, cells of the immune system are unable to respond to hormonal control, and consequently, produce levels of inflammation that promote disease. Because inflammation plays a role in many diseases such as cardiovascular, asthma and autoimmune disorders, this model suggests why stress impacts them as well."

Another result of the high cortisol levels associated with a stress response is food cravings. For women, those cravings typically tend to be strongest for carbs, especially sweet foods. We eat them seeking to feel better, but the more of them we eat, the worse our mood gets. As if that weren't bad enough, the cortisol then makes more trouble for us, triggering an enzyme in our fat cells that converts cortisone to more cortisol. Since our visceral fat cells (the ones in our abdomen, packed around our vital organs) have more of these enzymes than the subcutaneous fat cells (the ones on our thighs and butts, for example), stress causes many women to accumulate more belly fat. Some research has found that these belly fat cells, which have been linked to a greater risk for heart disease and diabetes, have four times as many cortisol receptors as regular fat cells.

I completely understand the scenario. You are up all night working or worrying about some difficult life circumstance, not eating properly, and struggling to just stay afloat emotionally. We all experience this kind of stress from time to time. But a consistent dose of this fight or flight response compromises your immune system and leaves you wide open to disease. I get it. My life has certainly not been easy, and I had to learn new coping skills when my world came crashing down around me.

After my diagnosis, my stress levels were through the roof. I was in a constant state of panic and despair. I found that listening to a soothing voice guiding me into a state of peace was healing and made significant changes in my mood and pain levels. This is called guided meditation, and it has been proven effective in reducing stress levels and increasing overall positive mental outlook.

There are times when we may need to seek professional help. Many of us find it difficult to admit that we can't handle a situation alone. We may find it uncomfortable to expose our vulnerable sides, or believe we should be able to handle our crises on our own. I found that having an objective, trained professional to help me work through my challenges was very comforting. It's ok to ask for help. Far from being a weakness, it is a sign of wisdom and strength to recognize and take care of your needs.

In addition to making time for meditation and getting extra help when we need it, we can also support our health by choosing foods that can help relieve stress.

FOODS THAT CAN HELP RELIEVE STRESS

Berries—anthocyanins that give blueberries and black-berries their deep color contain antioxidants that aid your brain in the production of dopamine, a chemical that is critical to coordination, memory function, and your mood.

Dark leafy greens—rich in folate, which helps your body produce mood-regulating neurotransmitters, including serotonin and dopamine.

Avocado—this superfruit will help eliminate stress eating by satisfying your hunger.

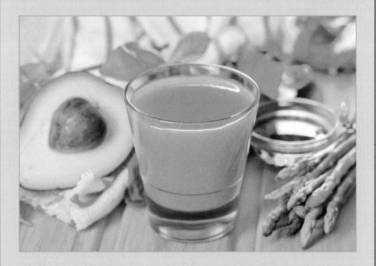

Asparagus—also rich in folate. Add them to your salads, steam, or broil them. They are also great grilled.

Banana—this low-calorie, naturally sweet fruit contains serotonin for relaxation as well as 30 percent of your daily allowance of vitamin B6.

Garlic—contains powerful antioxidants that neutralize free radicals that damage our cells. Garlic is helpful in warding off heart disease, cancer, and colds.

Green tea—contains theanine. Helps protect against some types of cancer. Theanine boosts mental performance. Green tea contains caffeine but can be found naturally decaffeinated as well.

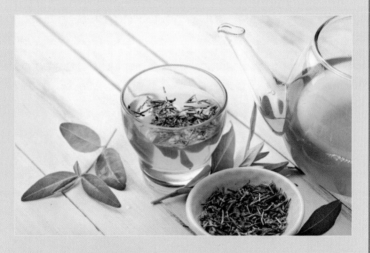

Oatmeal—a complex carbohydrate that causes your brain to produce serotonin that relaxes you.

Oranges—great source of vitamin C, an effective stress reliever.

Raisins—contain fiber and potassium. The polyphenols in raisins are effective in maintaining heart health and lowering blood pressure.

Walnuts—contain essential omega-3 fatty acid. Not only will they aid in reducing stress but will also improve your brainpower.

CHAPTER 8

Move Your Body for Good Health

I have exercised throughout my life and have always tried to stay in shape. Since my diagnosis of multiple sclerosis, I have found it very challenging to find a way to exercise without causing inflammation that can, at times, put pressure on my nerves and cause me pain. For that reason, I take things slowly and pay attention to how my body feels when exercising. If it hurts, I stop. Your body will tell you when it's too much. The secret is to learn to listen to it. And if the term "exercise" is intimidating, don't use it. Just make it your mission to move your body each day.

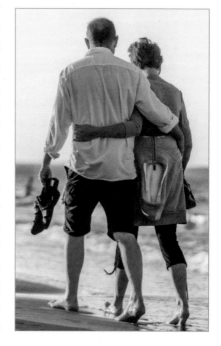

I learned that walking was a safe and effective way for me to move my body. I am blessed to have a dear friend who is my walking partner. We keep each other motivated to walk at least three times a week. When the weather does not cooperate, we walk the malls and motivate each other not to stop and spend money! Today I am walking an average of twenty miles each week.

There is probably someone in your circle of acquaintances who would love to start walking regularly but just hasn't committed to making it happen. Ask around. Let it be known that you are looking for a walking buddy—you may be surprised at the responses you will receive. You might be the reason another person starts their own journey toward better health.

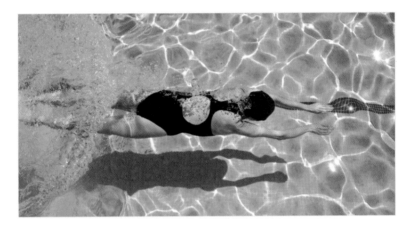

I have also found that swimming and pool aerobics are great forms of exercise for me, as well as gentle yoga. Yoga helps me stretch safely to maintain flexibility and alleviate muscle spasms. If you have MS, beware of Hot Yoga, as overheating exacerbates numbness and weakness. For toning and to maintain bone density, I enjoy lifting light weights.

Physical and occupational therapies have been very helpful to cope with the challenges of my disease. Physical therapy has helped me rebuild core muscles, relieve pain, and continue to improve my condition. In addition to teaching me how to relax, occupational therapy has taught me safe ways to move my body, sit, stand, and work at a computer correctly.

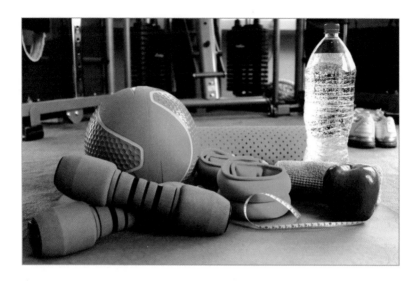

Each of us is unique with our own various challenges when it comes to exercise. Start out slowly and experiment with what feels best to you. The local gym after New Year's is a prime example of why this is so crucial. Fitness classes are overflowing, and it's hard to find an open piece of exercise equipment in January. But by March, classes are back to their usual sizes,

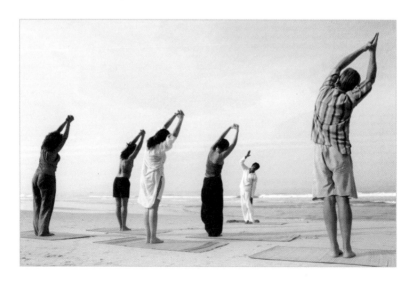

and you can easily find an empty treadmill or stair stepper. Why? People armed with a resolution to get fit and healthy hit the gym full force, don't listen to their bodies, choose exercises that don't fit them well, overdo it, and become discouraged. They may even go so hard they sustain an injury. They don't enjoy their workouts, and soon they give up on their resolution altogether. It's been said that the best exercise is the one you will do. Choose what you love—walking, dancing, bike riding, yoga, hiking. And keep your body moving.

Remember that before embarking on any new exercise program, be sure to check with your physician to insure that you are able to exercise safely. This is particularly important if you have any specific medical conditions or physical limitations. And don't forget to hydrate.

CHAPTER 9

Get Your Zzzs

A survey by the Harvard Women's Health Watch found that it is becoming more common for people to sleep less than six hours a night and that 75 percent of us experience sleep difficulties at least a few nights a week. We all have trouble falling or staying asleep sometimes. The problem occurs when this becomes chronic sleep loss. Studies show chronic sleep loss can contribute to weight gain, high blood pressure, and a compromised immune system. Not to mention the sluggishness and inability to be our best when we are functioning on a sleep deficit.

While many people turn to sleep medication for help, for many, this medication causes sleepwalking and other disturbing episodes that interfere with a good night's sleep. Another common side effect of sleep medication is memory lapses.

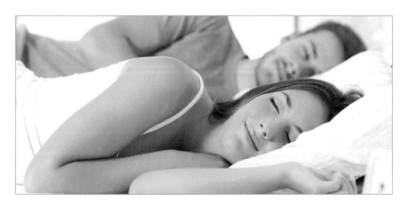

This is why it's important to educate yourself on all the possible side effects of the medications that you are prescribed. Ask your doctor or pharmacist to help you understand side effects and possible interactions with other medications and foods. If you find a link between your current medication and sleep difficulty, ask your doctor to switch you to alternative medication that may not interfere with your sleep patterns, but do not discontinue any medication without first checking with your doctor.

I found that many of the medications that I was prescribed for my MS made it difficult for me to get the rest that I desperately needed. After only three years of my initial diagnosis of MS, I was taking 18 pills per day. I was prescribed a sleep medication to help me sleep through the pain that I was experiencing. As time went on, the medications were not as effective and the dosages were increased. The sleep-inducing medication prescribed to me was the most difficult one for me to stop taking. I needed to re-establish my natural sleep rhythms, and it took time for my body to readjust.

As I added healthy, whole foods to my diet, my symptoms decreased and I was able to discontinue all medications. I cannot guarantee that these results will happen for you, nor am I encouraging anyone to stop taking medication that may be necessary. What I can say for sure is that eating to make your body as healthy as it can be is certainly an advantage if you are battling a disease.

To help you get your zzz's, consider eating foods that contain tryptophan, a sleep-enhancing amino acid that helps produce serotonin and melatonin which promote healthy sleep-wake cycles and help you fall asleep faster.

You can add these foods to your smoothies or juices or eat them at dinnertime to ease your way into a good night's sleep.

FOODS THAT CAN HELP YOU GET YOUR ZZZS

Yogurt helps your brain use tryptophan. Adding yogurt to an evening smoothie will help you to fall asleep.

Eat a small amount of **walnuts and/or almonds**. They contain tryptophan and magnesium. Be careful not to eat too many as they may increase weight gain. If you have diverticulitis, nuts may aggravate your stomach.

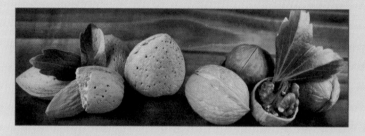

Lettuce contains lactucarium, which has sedative properties. Have a salad with your dinner. You can also try this brew from the book *Stealth Health:* Simmer three to four large lettuce leaves in a cup of water for 15 minutes. Remove from heat; add two sprigs of mint; and sip just before you go to bed. Consider adding this tea to a juice or smoothie in the evening after it has been brewed and cooled down.

Green leafy vegetables are loaded with calcium that helps the brain use tryptophan to manufacture melatonin.

Spinach, mustard greens, and kale are good options not only to eat, but also to add to your smoothies and juices for optimal health benefits.

Fish such as **tuna, halibut, and salmon** are high in vitamin B6 that your body requires to make melatonin and serotonin. When purchasing fish, choose wild caught or inquire about the feed given the fish if they are farm raised. Be sure to buy fish from responsible farming sources. Eat tuna in moderation as it contains increased levels of mercury.

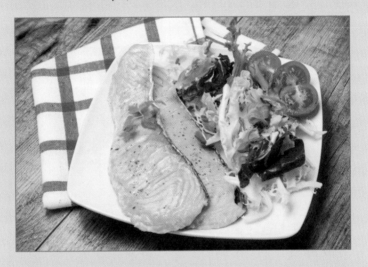

Organic tart cherry juice naturally boosts levels of melatonin. Drink a small glass about twenty minutes before going to bed.

Chamomile tea contains glycine that relaxes your nerves and muscles and acts like a mild sedative.

An Australian study found that drinking a cup of **passion fruit tea** one hour before bed helped people sleep more soundly. Researchers believe that Harman alkaloids, chemicals found in high levels in the passion fruit flower, act on your nervous system to make you tired.

CHAPTER 10

Energize!

When I ask people what health goals are most important to them, one of the most frequent answers I receive is, "I want to have more energy." There are so many factors that affect our energy levels.

In order to have more energy, we must be in good health. And good health is all about homeostasis, or balance. It's the yin and yang in life. You can eat the healthiest diet in the world, but if your personal life is unhappy, you are out of balance. Perhaps a significant relationship in your life is failing, your job is not fulfilling or your spiritual life is lacking substance. These situations can threaten the balance in our lives and zap us of energy.

Searching your heart to find what is blocking you from living a happy life is a first step to wellness. In addition, supporting your body during tough times is key to providing your immune system with the tools it needs to succeed in protecting you from illness and maintaining your energy levels.

Many of us Americans are addicted to processed and sugary foods containing few nutrients. These foods are the opposite of truly energizing. These sugars enter our bloodstream quickly, giving us a boost in energy, but that boost is short-lived and leaves us feeling tired and depleted. Examples of simple carbohydrates are shown on the next page.

SIMPLE CARBOHYDRATES

- High fructose corn syrup

- Corn syrup

- Breads, pasta, and baked goods made with white flour

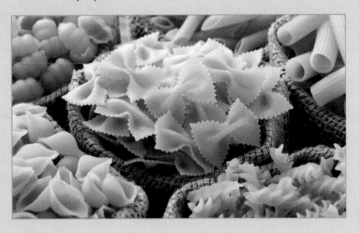

- Candy

- Cake

- Fruit juice

- Soda pop

- Most packaged cereals

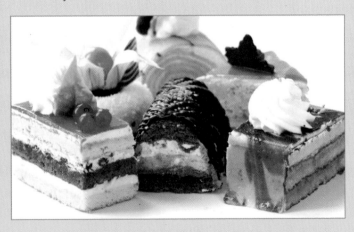

To avoid that dip in energy, watch out for foods that contain sugar, sucrose, fructose, corn syrup, white flour, or "wheat" flour and enriched flours. When you read a label, ingredients are listed in order of how much of it is contained in the product. So if sugar or corn syrup is listed near the top, this is not a food you want to consume for sustained energy.

Instead, choose foods that have not been highly processed or refined. Swap that glass of juice for a piece of fresh organic fruit; turn down that white bread in favor of organic whole grain bread. These are considered complex carbohydrates, and they are high in fiber and nutrients that improve digestion. Complex carbohydrates enter your bloodstream slowly, stabilize blood sugar, and provide you with longer lasting energy and better health. Some examples of complex carbohydrates are shown on the following page.

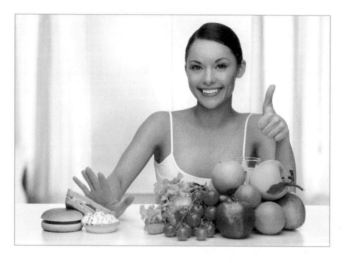

Caring for your body is much like maintaining your automobile. You need to use the correct fuel for optimal performance and provide it with routine maintenance. The big difference, of course, is that you can trade in your car but not your body. Be good to it and it will provide you with the energy you need.

COMPLEX CARBOHYDRATES

- Apples
- Pears
- Plums
- Strawberries
- Oranges

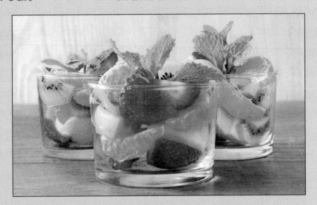

- Artichokes
- Asparagus
- Broccoli
- Navy beans
- Carrots
- Brown rice
- Lentils
- Yams (sweet potatoes)
- Oatmeal
- Multi grain bread

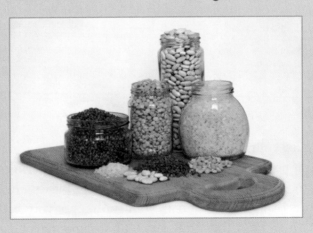

CHAPTER 11

Here's to Juices and Smoothies

To borrow a sentiment from an old country song—I was a juice and smoothie fan when juices and smoothies weren't cool. Think back a few years ago. How difficult was it to find a juice or smoothie bar in your neighborhood? Just one or two main franchises even existed. These days, anyone craving a fresh-squeezed green juice or a citrus smoothie can find a plethora of places to pack in the veggie goodness. Why the surge in popularity? Because lots of folks are getting serious about losing weight, regaining their energy, and living overall healthier lives. Juices and smoothies are a quick, delicious way to help achieve those goals.

Drinking your veggies is a quick and easy way to get your daily five servings of fresh vegetables and three servings of fresh fruit recommended by the United States Cancer Institute. And it's a way to tap into another key motivator for most folks—variety. We get bored of eating the same things all the time. Drinking your greens and veggies in healthy juices and smoothies adds variety to your diet. There is an endless number of sweet, savory, salty, and tart ingredients you can experiment with. So you will always be encouraged as you discover favorite new flavor combinations.

As we mentioned earlier, it's not always easy to get our children to eat the fruits and veggies their growing bodies need. Juices and smoothies are a perfect way to camouflage the "green things" and make them taste great. Why not show our kids that making healthy choices can be fun?

Smoothies contain fiber from fruits and vegetables that will fill you up and contribute to healthy digestion. Juicing eliminates the fiber, but the juice is packed with easily digestible nutrients—a significant benefit for those who are not well and need to add key vitamins, minerals, nutrients, and enzymes to their diets while not taxing the digestive system.

When choosing ingredients for your juices and smoothies, it is important that you use healthy options. Beware of adding too many fruits to your juices and smoothies as they contain natural sugars that can spike your insulin levels and can also be responsible for weight gain.

Don't be afraid to experiment by adding ingredients like cacao, chia seeds, or coconut oil to enhance the benefits of your smoothie or juice. Add green stevia to sweeten, aloe vera to soothe your stomach, or apple cider vinegar to relieve sore throats and decrease congestion. There are endless choices you can make to change up your recipes and receive the optimal benefits of drinking for your health.

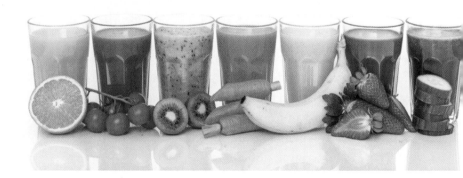

CHAPTER 12

Blender, Juicer— Or Both?

Smoothies and juices make it easy to incorporate lots of healthy fruits and vegetables into your daily routine. Let's talk about what you will need to make your own smoothies or juices at home.

Smoothies are made in powerful blending machines that make it possible to include many ingredients into your smoothies that you would be unable to use with a juicer. Some of those ingredients are nutritious nuts, grains, seeds, herbs, or supplements. Smoothies maintain the fiber content of the fruits and

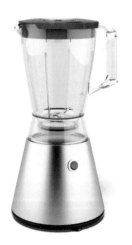
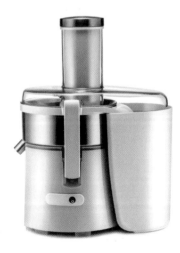

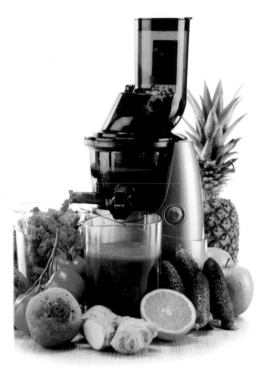

vegetables so you use less produce. They are thickly textured and more filling than juice. I make my smoothies in a Vitamix, a very powerful machine that not only makes great smoothies, but also produces delicious hot soups —perfect on a chilly fall day.

Juices are made in masticating or centrifugal machines that separate the pulp from the juice. Juicers eliminate most of the fiber but preserve nutrients and enzymes as they generate less heat and friction.

Juices are lightly textured and easily digested and provide a storehouse of valuable nutrients to persons recovering from surgery or major illnesses. Juicing uses more produce and ingredients than smoothies making it a more expensive option. If cost of a juicer is prohibitive, you can make your own in a regular blender, but it is time-consuming and messy because you will need to strain the fiber through a sieve, cheesecloth, or other straining device.

When shopping for a blending machine for smoothies or juices, choose one with a powerful motor and that is easy to clean. Cleaning a blending machine is quick and easy—rinse, add water and dish soap, blend a few seconds, then hit it with a scrub brush for safe measure. Rinse again and you're done. Or just throw the whole thing in the dishwasher. Juicers require a bit more work to clean the pulp that has been extracted from the fruits and veggies. So if you want to be able to throw together a quick healthy drink in the morning and head off to work, you may want to choose a blender over a juicer.

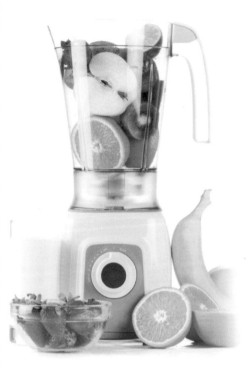

For either a blender or a juicer, having a large opening to add whole fruits and vegetables is helpful. Consider the amount of liquid that can be extracted so that you don't have to stop and clean the machine repeatedly. Check out the warranty on the motor and parts, and look for a 5- to 10-year plan.

Prior to purchasing a blending machine, sample some smoothies and juices to determine what your preference would be. A blender or juicer is a substantial investment, so you want to make sure you will use it. If you love both juices and smoothies, and cost is not an issue, by all means purchase both. What a treat to have your own fresh, healthy juices and smoothies any time!

Both juices and smoothies provide amazing health benefits but only if you actually drink them. The bottom line is to choose the type of machine that suits you and that you will use regularly in order to get those healthy fruits and veggies working for you. The key is to make it an enjoyable experience that will bring you healthy rewards.

CHAPTER 13

Tips for Making Smoothies and Juices

When you begin your adventure into making smoothies and juices, keep them simple. For some, green juices and smoothies are an acquired taste. Adding too many greens may taste unpleasant to you at first. Feel free to add an extra apple or other sweet fruit or vegetable of your choice. As you adjust to drinking your juices and smoothies, begin to lessen the amount of these sweeter ingredients so that you get the benefit of the greens and do not consume as much sugar. Although the sugar in sweeter fruits and vegetables is from a natural source, it can contribute to weight gain, cravings, and raised levels of insulin in your body. A good guideline for juicing and blending is—sweetness in moderation.

I like to think of making juices and smoothies as a refrigerator cleanout. Don't let valuable fruits, greens, and vegetables sitting in your fridge go to waste. There are no strict rules for creating these healthy drinks other than to try different ingredients and enjoy your journey to better health.

Try These in Your Juices and Smoothies

Berries are packed with antioxidants that can help prevent oxidative stress which is linked to chronic diseases and aging.

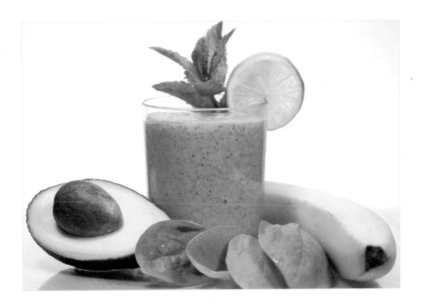

Consuming berries is a flavorful way to satisfy your sweet tooth without the crash of processed sugar. Use frozen organic berries when fresh are not available.

For those who are sensitive to dairy, use juice or rice, nut, or soy milks. Other great additions are green tea, mint tea, coconut oil, and organic fruit juices.

If your juice or smoothie is too sweet, try adding lemon juice, one tablespoon at a time, until it's just right. If your juice or smoothie is too sour, try adding chopped sweet fruit, such as an apple, grapes, or pineapple.

Kiwis contain more immunity boosting vitamin C per serving than oranges do. If you are getting a cold, add kiwi to your smoothies and juices. Peel before using.

Although bananas are great in smoothies, they do not juice well. They are a good source of potassium and help curb hunger.

One cup of spinach provides 40 percent of our daily require-
ment of magnesium, a mineral shown to lower stress levels.
Headaches, general fatigue, and irritability indicate that your
magnesium levels may be deficient.

Mustard, turnip, and collard greens are excellent sources of
calcium. Calcium helps our brains to produce tryptophan that
releases melatonin, known to increase drowsiness and sustain
REM sleep.

Papaya is an excellent source of vitamin C and may also
reduce absorption of cancer-causing nitrosamines. There is
some evidence that foods like papaya that are high in folic acid
may prevent certain types of cancer. Papaya is also an effective
way to settle upset stomachs and acid indigestion.

Add avocados to your smoothies for a good source of DHA
Omega-3 fatty acids and healthy fat that will improve heart
health and overall brain health as well as provide anti-aging
benefits. Healthy fats like those in avocados protect your organs,
keep your body warm, and help to absorb nutrients. While bad
fats—saturated and trans fats—can clog your arteries and raise
the bad cholesterol levels (LDL) in your blood, good fats—

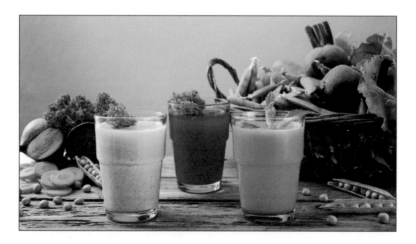

monounsaturated and polyunsaturated fats—can lower bad cholesterol levels and are a beneficial addition to a healthy diet.

Pineapple contains bromelain that has anti-inflammatory properties. It is thought to ease arthritis pain and is good for digestive health, cancer prevention, and acne.

Matcha Green Tea is a finely ground, bright emerald green tea powder. It is prepared from a high-quality shade-grown leaf known as tencha. These tea bushes are sheltered to avoid exposure of direct sunlight, which reduces the pace of photosynthesis and slows down the growth of the plants. Drinking matcha tea improves mental alertness and clarity as well as aiding in stronger immune defense and detoxification. Polyphenol- and catechin-rich matcha promotes relaxation and is beneficial for prevention and treatment of various medical conditions including bacterial, fungal and viral infections, cancer and type-2 diabetes. It also assists in maintaining cardiovascular health and gastrointestinal health.

Dragon fruit, or pitaya, is loaded with protein, iron, and vitamin C. They are especially rich in antioxidants, and the fruit peel may inhibit the growth of certain cancers. The seeds of the fruit are similar to kiwi seeds and are edible.

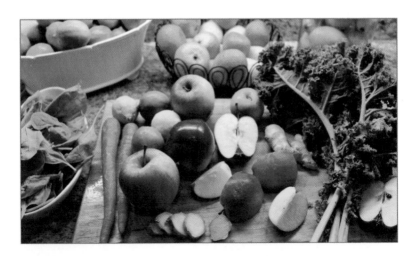

CHAPTER 14

Delicious, Nutritious Smoothie Recipes

Are you ready to make yourself a nice, refreshing smoothie? First, make sure your produce is washed well, and remember to use organic whenever possible. You will find in the recipes that follow, I have omitted certain repetitive steps or directions that are common to all blending recipes. For example, for all smoothie recipes, add liquid first before the remainder of the ingredients. I have listed some of my preferences for these liquids, but I encourage you to search out healthy alternatives that you would enjoy most.

Before blending, make sure your lid is on securely to prevent a mess on your counter—I say this from experience. Blend slowly at first, gradually increasing the speed until smooth.

If you find your smoothie too thick, add more liquid as desired. Adding ice cubes or frozen fruits and vegetables will give you a nice, cool, frosty drink. For a creamier smoothie, add organic yogurt, avocado, or banana. For added benefit, consider adding healthy plant-based protein powder, cacao, maca, goji berries, fish oil, coconut oil, flax seeds, chia seeds, green tea, or aloe. Add green stevia, honey, or maple syrup if more sweetness is desired.

NOTE: If you are pregnant or nursing, many holistic natural health practitioners advise eliminating parsley from your diet due to its potential affect on the uterus during pregnancy and also on milk production during lactation.

BERRY GREEN SMOOTHIE

Anti-inflammatory

1 rib of celery

1 cup of kale

1/2 cup of strawberries, hulled

half lime, peeled

1 cup coconut water

YUMMY TUMMY

Anti-inflammatory

1/2 cup baby spinach

1/2 cup frozen mangos

1/2 cup fresh papaya

1/4 cup walnuts

1/2 inch fresh ginger root

1/2 inch fresh turmeric root

1/2 tsp. ground cinnamon

1 cup unsweetened coconut milk

If you do not have a Vitamix or similar processor, grind walnuts prior to adding to your machine.

PAPAYA PINEAPPLE PASSION

Digestive aid

¼ cup of papaya, chopped

2 cups fresh pineapple, chopped

1 cup almond milk

½ cup freshly squeezed organic orange juice

¼ cup organic coconut milk

½ tsp. freshly squeezed lime juice

½ tsp. maple syrup

Combine all ingredients in blender or processor. Blend until smooth.

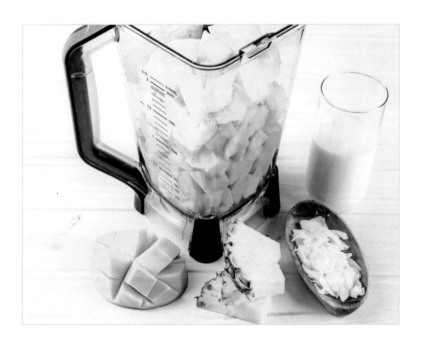

BANANA POWER

Great for energy and endurance

1 cup celery, chopped

$\frac{1}{4}$ cup cashews

2 bananas

$\frac{1}{4}$ cup plant-based protein powder

$1\frac{1}{2}$ tsp. spirulina

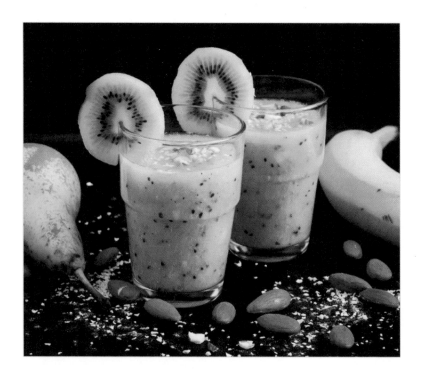

BYE BYE BELLY ACHE

Aids in digestion

1 cup organic baby spinach

1 cucumber, peeled

1 kiwi fruit, peeled

1 cup watermelon, rind removed

Aloe vera gel; discard tough outer leaf

AVOCADO DREAM

Great way to add healthy fat to your diet

1 avocado

1 banana

3 dates, pitted

1 Tbsp. freshly squeezed lemon juice

1 cup organic baby kale

1 cup almond or rice milk

Add a few ice cubes if you prefer this chilled.

SWEET DREAMS

Sleep inducing

1 kiwi, peeled

1 frozen banana

½ cup uncooked oats

2 cups kale

1 Tbsp. honey

1 Tbsp. almond butter

½ cup almond or rice milk

Add milk and oats to your machine. Blend into paste; add remainder of ingredients and blend again until smooth. Add more liquid if desired.

BE WELL

Immunity boost

1 cup freshly squeezed orange juice

1 carrot, peeled and chopped

2 handfuls Swiss chard

1 cup strawberries, fresh or frozen

1 Tbsp. organic raw pumpkin seeds

1 Tbsp. organic raw sunflower seeds

BERRY GOOD BONES

Helps prevent bone loss

1 cup coconut water

1 banana

1/2 cup organic blueberries,
fresh or frozen

1/2 cup organic raspberries,
fresh or frozen

1/4 cup wheat bran

10 organic raw cashews

2 Tbsp. raw cacao

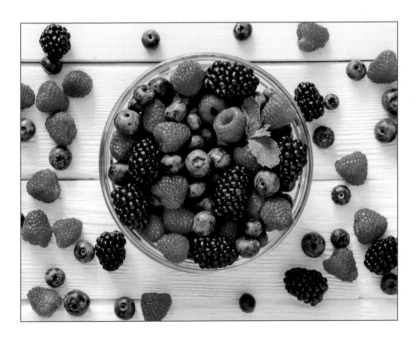

MS BUSTER

Smoothie for multiple sclerosis

1 cup organic plain yogurt

1½ tsp. chia seeds

1½ tsp. flaxseeds

¾ cup organic strawberries
or blueberries, fresh or frozen

1 handful mint leaves

1-inch slice fresh ginger,
peeled and chopped

½ tsp. cinnamon

1 cup of ice cubes

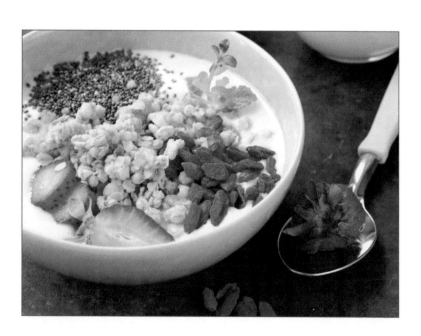

BERRY YOUNG

Anti-aging

1 1/2 cup coconut water

1/2 cup fresh or frozen
organic blueberries

1/2 cup fresh or frozen
organic raspberries

2 handfuls of greens
such as spinach or chard

REFRESH AND CLEAN

Detox

2 handfuls spinach

1 large fresh squeezed orange

2 bananas

1/2 lemon, peeled and seeded

1/2 lime, peeled and seeded

1/2 cup ice

BEAUTIFY ME

Beautiful hair, skin and nails

1 cup coconut water

2 handfuls baby kale

1 banana

1½ cups mango, cut into chunks,
fresh or frozen

THE ELVIS—PB AND BANANA

2 Servings

1 banana

1 cup almond milk

1 cup kale, chopped

2 Tbsp. peanut butter, organic

¼ tsp. ground cinnamon

⅛ tsp. nutmeg

Add 1 banana, nut milk, kale, peanut butter, ground
cinnamon, nutmeg and ½ cup ice in a blender and
blend until smooth.

*For a cooler smoothie, freeze the banana prior to blending.

BERRY BLUE SMOOTHIE

2 Servings

1½ cups fresh (or frozen, thawed)
organic blueberries

½ cup unsweetened coconut milk

1 Tbsp. fresh mint leaves

1 tsp. fresh lime juice

1 tsp. local honey or raw honey*

Blend blueberries, coconut milk, lime juice, mint, honey
and 1 cup of ice until smooth.

---

*Do not feed honey to children under 2 years of age.

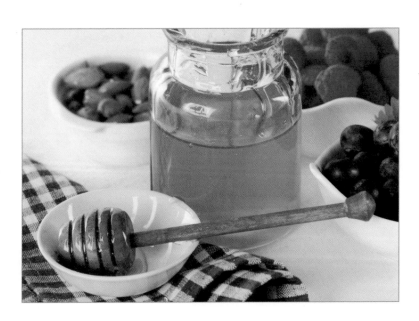

RAZZMATAZZ SMOOTHIE

2 Servings

½ cup (packed) flat-leaf parsley
(leaves and stems)

4 kale leaves, remove stems

1 cup frozen organic raspberries

1 banana, sliced

Blend all ingredients with 1 cup water until smooth
(add more water to reach desired thickness).

GREEN TEA SMOOTHIE

1 cup green tea,
brewed and chilled

1 Granny Smith apple,
cored and seeded

½ cup baby kale

1 Tbsp. plain organic Greek yogurt

MATCHA FOR HEALTH

1 tsp.green tea matcha powder*

1 cup coconut milk

1/2 cup frozen blueberries

Blend the ingredients until they are smooth.

---

*Green tea matcha or maccha can be found in organic food stores as well as in Asian markets. (See chapter 13 for more information)

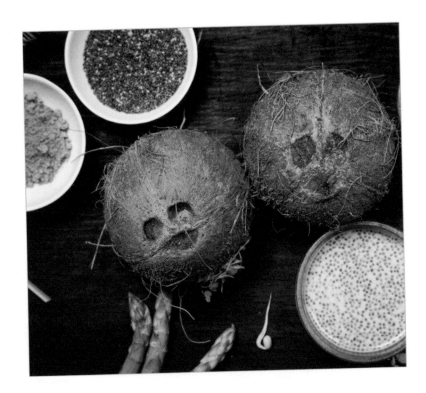

MANGO TANGO

1 banana, peeled and frozen

½ cup mango, peeled and seeded

½ avocado

1 cup baby organic spinach

1¼ cups vanilla flavored almond milk

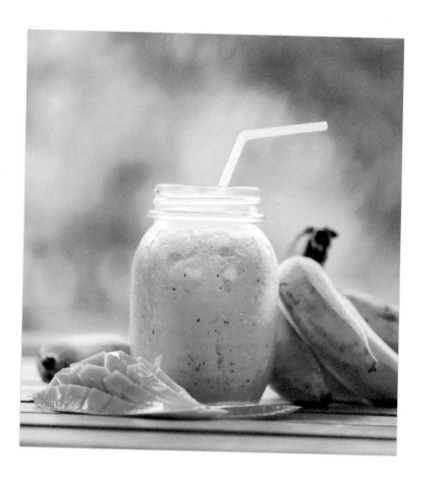

STRAWBERRY COCONUT SMOOTHIE

1½ cups rice milk

1 cup strawberries, hulled

1 Tbsp. coconut oil

1 banana

1 Tbsp. local honey

Blend until smooth. Sprinkle with cinnamon, if desired

BERRY COCONUT POWER SMOOTHIE

½ cup yogurt

½ cup strawberries

1 banana, peeled and frozen

1 Tbsp. coconut oil

1 scoop of chocolate plant-based protein powder

2 cups spring water

APPLE GRAPE SMOOTHIE

1 cup organic red seedless grapes*

1 banana, sliced

½ green apple,
cored and quartered

1½ cups fresh spinach leaves

---

*Seedless grapes are great frozen as a snack. You can also use frozen grapes in your smoothies to cool your drink.

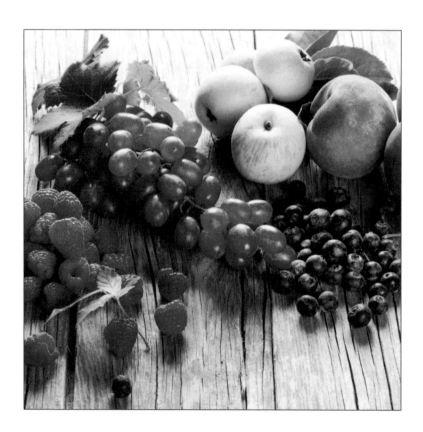

BLUE BASIL SMOOTHIE

1 cup blueberries,
fresh or frozen

1 banana, frozen

$1/4$ cup fresh basil leaves

$1/2$ cup organic baby spinach leaves

2 cups organic almond milk

BANOCCOLI SMOOTHIE

Cancer prevention

$1\,1/2$ cups coconut milk

1 banana, peeled

1 cup broccoli florets

1 tsp. ground cinnamon

1 Tbsp. raw honey

ALLSTAR SMOOTHIE

Loaded with vitamin C

½ starfruit, seeds removed*

½ cup pineapple, peeled, cored and cubed

1 apple, cored and seeded

1 cup kale, stems removed and chopped

1 small banana, peeled and sliced

8 oz. coconut water

Put coconut water into the blender. Add the remaining ingredients and blend until smooth.

---

*Starfruit, also known as carambola, may interact with some medications and should not be consumed by those with kidney disease. Please consult with your physician prior to using. You may eliminate the starfruit, if desired.

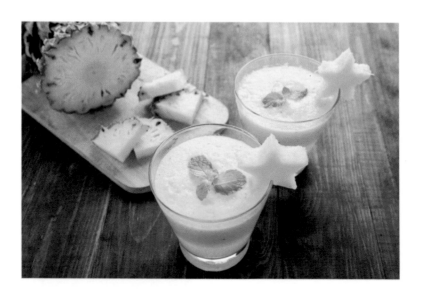

CHAPTER 15

Tasty Juice Recipes

Drink your fresh juice on an empty stomach. This allows the vitamins and minerals in the juice to go straight into your bloodstream so that your body can quickly absorb the nutrients. Juicing on a full stomach can result in heartburn or other digestive issues. A general rule of thumb is to wait at least two hours after a meal to drink a green juice, and wait 20 minutes after drinking a green juice to consume a meal.

For optimum health benefits, drink your juice within 15 minutes after it's been made. As soon as freshly made green juice is exposed to air, its live enzymes begin to degrade, decreasing the nutritional benefits of the juice. The live enzymes of a fresh juice provide immediate energy; stored juice will not.

If you really want to store your juice, keep it refrigerated at all times before consuming. Store in an airtight container filled to the top for no more than 24–36 hours. A press juicer eliminates air in the juice so that it can be stored up to 72 hours. This is important to remember when you buy pre-made, raw, unpasteurized juice. As soon as the juice becomes warm, harmful bacteria can begin to grow and affect your health.

Beware of using too many high-sugar fruits and vegetables in your green juice. Sweet fruits and vegetables such watermelon, apples, pears, mangos, beets, and carrots are nutritious when eaten whole. But as we've already discussed, it's easy to pack too much sweetness into a smoothie. Focus on the greens.

Help your body to digest juice by swishing it in your mouth for a couple of seconds before swallowing. This releases saliva that contains important digestive enzymes which are crucial in delivering key nutrients to your cells and provide the optimal health benefit of the juice.

Rotate your greens such as kale, chard, spinach, mustard greens, arugula, etc., each week to prevent buildup of oxalic acid that can affect the thyroid gland. Adding a variety of greens will provide a balanced amount of different vitamins and minerals for your body.

There is no better way to fuel your body with the powerful nutrients inside green vegetables than to juice them. Because our soil is nutritionally depleted due to the use of pesticides, genetically modified seeds, and conventional farming practices, the level of vitamins and minerals once abundant in our crops has been decreased dramatically. Today, eating fruits and vegetables does not provide the same amount of nutrition as it did years ago. Juicing is an effective way to get the most benefit without having to eat crazy amounts of fruits and vegetables to make up for the lack of nutrients. Juicing is beneficial for those battling disease or as preventive medicine to avoid disease by reducing the amount of energy your body uses for digestion. This gives your cells a chance to repair and rebuild.

Don't wait until you are sick or trying to recover to add healthy juice to your diet. Take care of your body and it will take care of you. Juicing provides it with the tools it needs to keep you healthy and energized.

JUICING MACHINE TIPS

Some ingredients such as nuts and seeds do not juice well and may clog your juicer. Read your machine's instructions for guidelines of preferred foods for your specific juicer.

Clean your juicer well after each use. Use a brush (they usually come with the juicing machine) to make sure all pulp residue is removed from the filter of the machine. Check your machine guide for specific cleaning instruction. Most parts are dishwasher safe, which is helpful for killing any remaining bacteria.

Some juicers have a fiber separator that can be removed if you prefer to have some of the fiber remain in your juice. The separator should be used if you prefer pure juice or if you are having a difficult time digesting foods due to stomach issues or illness.

Be sure that the cover of the juicer is securely attached prior to juicing.

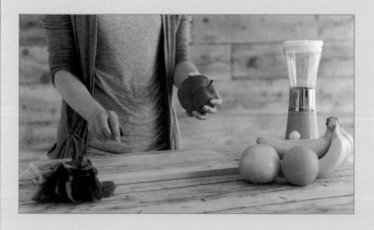

THE GUARDIAN

Immune booster

2 Granny Smith apples,
seeded and cored

4 celery stalks

1 cucumber

6 kale leaves

$\frac{1}{2}$ lemon, peeled

1-inch piece ginger, peeled

1 oz. wheatgrass juice,
fresh if possible

Wheatgrass juice can be found in your organic grocer's frozen food section if fresh is unavailable. Use one or two cubes as desired.

PEP IN YOUR STEP

Energy

2 green apples, seeded and cored

1 Tbsp. honey, local if possible

$\frac{1}{2}$ lemon, peeled

1 cup pure spring water

SWEET ENERGY

Perfect beginner juice

1 apple, seeded and cored

1 large carrot

1 large beetroot

1 bunch of kale, slightly chopped

Add pure spring water or
carrot juice if needed.

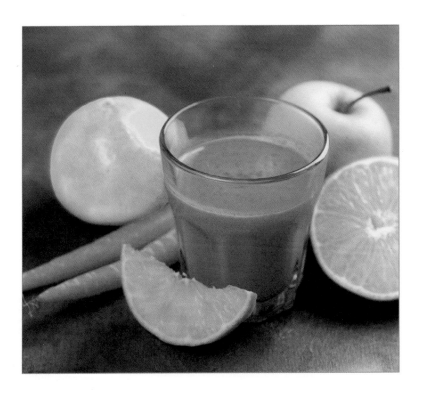

REV UP YOUR ENGINE

Heart health and energy

1 grapefruit, peeled*

5 celery stalks

1 bunch of kale

1 Red Delicious apple,
seeded and cored

---

*Grapefruit may interact with certain statin medications and may affect its efficacy. Consult with your physician prior to ingesting grapefruit or its juice.

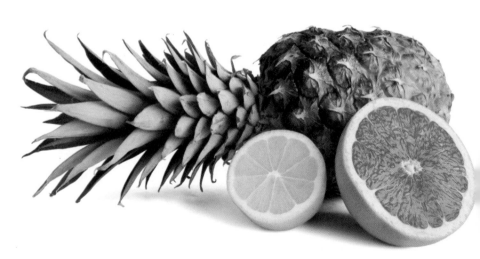

CALM AND DIGEST

Anti-inflammatory

1 cup fresh pineapple,
peeled and chopped

1 pear, seeded and cored

$1/2$ cup fresh mint leaves,
stems included

$1/2$ cucumber

SIMPLY GREEN JUICE

Detox and strengthen

1 bunch of kale, chopped

1 cucumber

1 parsley sprig
(omit if pregnant or nursing)

$1/2$ lemon, peeled

1 Granny Smith apple,
seeded and cored

1 cup spinach

2-inch piece of aloe, peeled

Aloe vera juice can be added
for desired consistency.

YEAST BE GONE

Juice for candida

1 Granny Smith apple,
cored

1 head of broccoli,
stems included

3 celery stalks

1 garlic clove, peeled

$1/2$ small onion, peeled

HEALTHY HEART

1 red apple, medium, cored

$1/2$ cucumber

4 celery stalks

2 cups green grapes

1 cup pomegranate seeds

4 cups spinach

Yields approximately 4 cups of juice.

GRANT ME IMMUNITY

Boost immune system

2 red apples, peeled and cored

2 red beets

1 orange, peeled

2 cloves of garlic, peeled

1 handful of Swiss chard leaves

1 one inch piece of ginger root, peeled

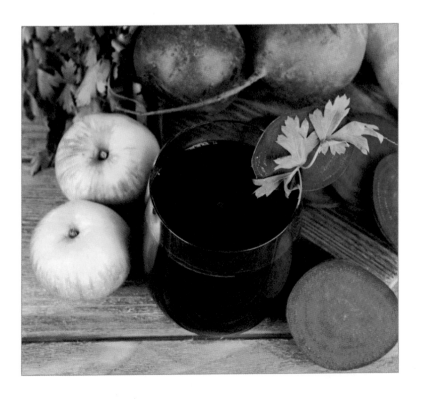

MANGO MAGIC

Energy and vitality

1 mango, seeded and peeled

½ cup wheatgrass*

3 romaine lettuce leaves

1 large kale leaf

1 pear, seeded and cored

1 apple, seeded and cored

1 cucumber

---

*Wheatgrass juice can be purchased in the frozen foods section of most health food stores. If using frozen, add 1 or 2 cubes as desired.

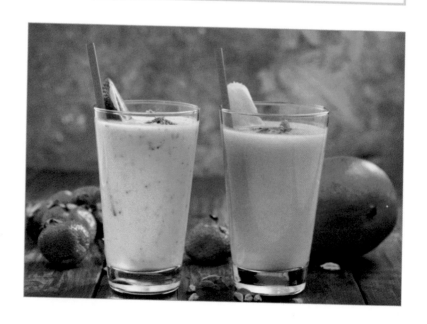

POWER JUICE

Energy boost

2 red apples, medium,
cored

3 carrots

3 celery stalks

1 1-inch piece of ginger root,
peeled

2 Bartlett pears, medium,
cored

1 2-inch piece of turmeric root

THE GREEN DRAGON

Healing for nerves

$\frac{1}{2}$ cup dragon fruit, peeled

5 large strawberries

2 cups fresh baby spinach

6 ounces coconut water

GREEN PAIN KILLER

Anti-inflammatory

2-inch piece of turmeric

5 romaine leaves

2 carrots

1 stalk celery

1 cucumber

1 lemon, peeled

Add turmeric, romaine, carrots, celery, lemon, and cucumber to juicer.

WATERMELON JUICE

Weight loss aid

$1/4$ medium sized watermelon, including rind*

1 medium cucumber

1 bunch of kale, including stems

1 lime, peeled

1 small orange, peeled

Slice the rind into strips. Add ingredients to juicer, alternating the softer ones with the more dense.

DRINK YOUR BROCCOLI

Weight loss, diabetes and heart disease

1 bunch of broccoli,
stalk and florets

2 organic red apples,
cored and seeded

2 lemons, peeled

1 cup baby spinach

2 stalks of celery

1 large cucumber

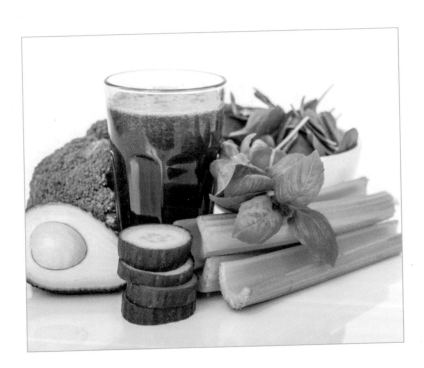

GREEN GIANT JUICE

Immune booster

1 red apple, cored and seeded

1 pear, cored and seeded

1 cucumber

1-inch piece fresh ginger root

1 cup arugula, firmly packed

$\frac{1}{2}$ cup fresh cilantro

$\frac{1}{2}$ cup fresh parsley

1 lemon, peeled

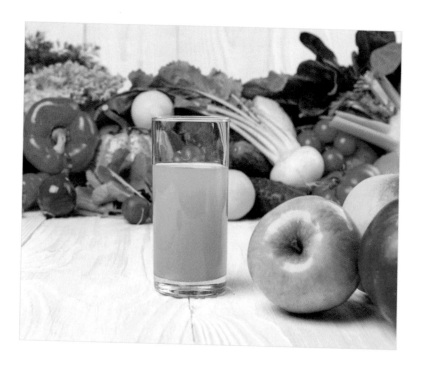

PINEAPPLE PAIN RELIEF

Anti-inflammatory; relief from menstrual pain

5 ribs of celery

1/2 bulb of fennel

1/2 small pineapple,
peeled and cut into chunks

1-inch ginger root

SALAD IN A GLASS

Vitamin C and digestion

4 romaine lettuce leaves,
chopped

1 large tomato,
cut into wedges

1 small organic red bell
pepper, sliced

1 large stalks celery,
trimmed

1 small carrot

1 cucumber

Ice, if desired.

GREEN CHIA JUICE

Good for digestion

1 large collard leaf

1 large kale leaf

1 green apple

1 cucumber

1 lemon, peeled

1 tsp. chia seeds*

---

*Soak chia seeds in water to soften prior to juicing.

HEALTHY WATERCRESS JUICE

High in vitamin K, great for bone health

1 bunch of watercress

1 zucchini

1 apple, cored and seeded

½ lemon, peeled

ASIAN PEAR JUICE

Blood, bone, and cardiovascular health

2 Asian pears,
cored and seeded

1 cup fresh basil, leaves and stems,
firmly packed

1 lemon, peeled

2 large celery stalks

Put basil leaves in juicer, follow with celery stalks, pears and lemon. Add ice, if desired.

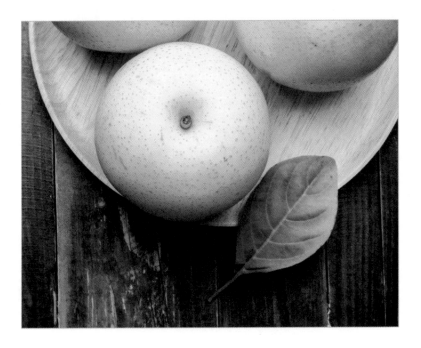

GOJI PINEAPPLE JUICE

Energy and health boost

¼ cup goji berries*

¼ fresh pineapple, peeled,
cored and cubed

1 large kale leaf, chopped

4 cups ice cubes

*Cover goji berries in spring water or your favorite juice. Let sit for 10 minutes prior to adding them into your juicer.

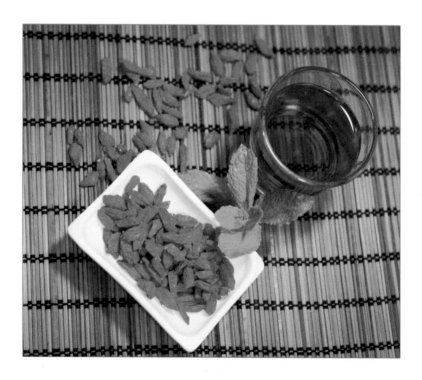

ISLAND GREEN JUICE

Anti-inflammatory

$1/2$ papaya

$1/2$ pineapple, peeled, cored and cubed

1 kiwi

3 cups watermelon, cubed

$1 1/2$ cups kale, firmly packed and chopped

1 cucumber

$1/2$ lemon, peeled

DANDY OF A JUICE

Boost immunity

$1/2$ cup dandelion greens, firmly packed

$1/2$ cup baby spinach leaves, firmly packed

6 apricots, pitted*

1 navel orange, peeled

1 small aloe vera leaf, peeled**

*If fresh apricots are not available, soak dried apricots in warm water until plump.

**You can substitute fresh aloe vera leaf with aloe vera juice if desired.

CANTALOUPE CLEANSE

Immune boost

$1/4$ cantaloupe, peeled and seeded

1 bunch watercress

1 large stalk celery

$1/2$ cup parsley

$1/2$ inch piece of ginger

$1/2$ lemon, peeled

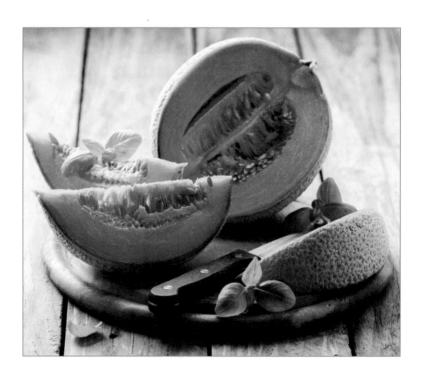

CHAPTER 16

Tempting Greens
for Your Plate

Smoothies and juices are a simple, versatile way to enjoy your fruits and veggies each day. Of course, we also need flavorful, nutritious options when it's time to sit down at the table for a traditional meal. Gathering around the table with family and friends is an important part of our lives. It is a time to enrich our lives with great conversation and healthy foods. I find it fulfilling to serve my family and friends a meal chock full of vitamins and nutrients that tastes great and keeps them in good health.

You can still reap all the healthy benefits of a smoothie or a juice while using your fork. You just have to be intentional about incorporating lots of greens into your recipes and choosing recipes that you really enjoy preparing and eating. When you choose your recipes wisely, you will actually find yourself looking forward to the process—shopping for your produce; cleaning, chopping and dicing; and finally, sitting down to a satisfying meal that features greens in the starring role.

There are limitless ways to prepare and enjoy nutritious greens—from green leafy salads, soups and stews, to tasty side dishes on your plate at breakfast, lunch, and dinner. Here are some of my favorites. Bon appetit!

SALADS

POMEGRANATE ARUGULA SALAD

Serves 4

6 cups baby arugula

1 pomegranate, seeded
*See hint below

1/4 purple onion, sliced thin

1/4 cup crumbled goat
cheese

1/4 cup toasted almonds,
sliced

Dressing:

1/4 cup pomegranate
molasses

2 Tbsp. honey,
local if possible

2 Tbsp. red wine vinegar

3/4 cup extra virgin
olive oil

Put salad ingredients into large salad bowl. Toss until well blended.

Whisk molasses, lemon juice, honey, and vinegar in a mixing bowl until combined. Slowly drizzle in olive oil while you whisk until emulsified. Season with salt and pepper.

Drizzle dressing over the salad mixture and toss.

---

* To seed pomegranate, cut fruit into quarters. Hold pomegranate over a bowl and hit the skin with a large spoon. The seeds will fall into the bowl.

FIELD GREEN SALAD WITH BERRIES

Serves 4–6

12 cups mixed field greens

1 cup red raspberries

1 cup blueberries

1 cup toasted pecans

3 oz. goat cheese

Dressing:

$\frac{1}{2}$ cup extra virgin olive oil

$\frac{1}{4}$ cup balsamic vinegar

Freshly ground black pepper

Salt to taste

Place greens in large salad bowl. Add berries and toasted pecans.

In a small bowl, whisk olive oil and vinegar until well blended.

Toss dressing into the greens and berries. Sprinkle roasted nuts over the salad. Cut chilled goat cheese into pieces and add to the bowl.

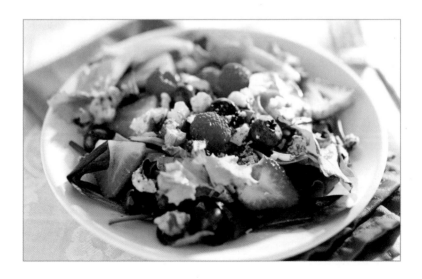

KALE AND AVOCADO CAESAR SALAD

Serves 4–6

5 anchovies, preserved in oil

2 small cloves of garlic, peeled and crushed

1 tsp. Dijon mustard

1 tsp. Worcestershire sauce

1 whole avocado, peeled and diced

Juice from $1/2$ lemon

$1/4$ cup extra virgin olive oil

$1/2$ cup mayonnaise

$1/2$ cup Parmesan, shredded

2 bunches of kale, ribs removed and sliced thin

Croutons:

3 cups cubed crusty bread

$1/2$ cup olive oil

1 large clove fresh garlic, minced

1 Tbsp. fresh parsley, finely chopped

Salt and pepper

Place anchovies, garlic, Worcestershire, and Dijon mustard into food processor. Pulse together until garlic is finely chopped. Add lemon juice, olive oil, and mayonnaise. Blend until smooth. Add small amounts water to mixture and pulse until desired consistency.

Transfer the dressing to a bowl; stir in the Parmesan. Cover with plastic wrap touching the surface of the dressing. Refrigerate.

Put prepared kale in a large bowl and sprinkle it with approximately $1/2$ tsp. of salt. Press the leaves and salt together with your hands for several minutes to allow salt to begin to soften the kale.

To make croutons:

Add 1 large clove garlic, minced and chopped fresh parsley to olive oil. Whisk until well blended.

Lightly brush the bread cubes with olive oil and place on baking sheet in a single layer. Bake in 350-degree oven until golden, about 10 minutes. Remove from oven and cool.

When ready to eat, toss the kale with desired amount of dressing. Top with croutons and avocado. Sprinkle with Parmesan cheese. Serve immediately.

ORANGE WATERCRESS SALAD

Serves 4–6

6 cups watercress

1 navel orange, peeled, skinned and separated into sections

1/2 Vidalia or sweet onion, sliced thin

1 avocado, peeled and sliced

1/2 cup sliced almonds, toasted

Dressing:

1/4 cup unseasoned rice vinegar

4 tsp. soy sauce (gluten free alternative is Tamari)

1 tsp. organic cane sugar (substitute agave nectar if desired)

3 Tbsp. olive oil

Whisk the dressing ingredients in a small bowl until well blended. Place the salad ingredients in bowl. Top with dressing and toss. Serve immediately.

COLORFUL CABBAGE SLAW

Serves 4–6

3 cups Napa cabbage, thinly sliced

3 cups red cabbage, thinly sliced

3 carrots, grated

4 scallions, thinly sliced including the green

1 can sliced water chestnuts, drained, rinsed

1/3 cup roasted peanuts, coarsely chopped

Dressing:

3 Tbsp. olive oil

2 Tbsp. Dijon mustard

1 Tbsp. agave nectar

2 Tbsp. rice wine vinegar

1 tsp. sesame oil

Whisk the dressing ingredients in a small bowl until well blended.

Toss salad ingredients together in a large bowl. Add dressing and toss to coat.

Serve immediately.

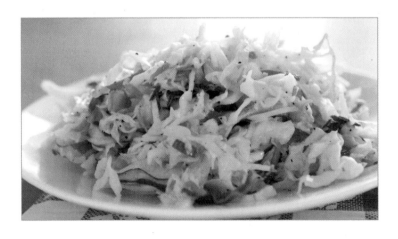

SOUPS

WHITE BEAN SOUP WITH TURNIP GREENS

1 20-oz. package Great Northern beans

1/2 large red onion, diced

2 stalks celery, diced

1 garlic clove, minced

1/2 tsp. oregano, dried

1/2 tsp. thyme, dried

1/2 tsp. black pepper

1 lb. cleaned, sliced turnip greens or greens of your choice

1/4 tsp. red pepper flakes

1 Tbsp. salt

2 fresh tomatoes, diced

1 bunch scallions, chopped

Put the beans in a large soup pot. Add water to cover the top of the beans. Add salt to water and bring beans to a rolling boil over high heat. Remove from the heat and let sit for one hour. Do not drain.

Place the beans and water back over high heat. Add the red onion, celery, garlic, herbs, pepper, turnip greens, and red pepper to the pot and bring to a boil. Cover the pot and reduce the heat.

Simmer an additional hour or until the beans are tender. Add salt and pepper to taste.

Ladle the soup into individual serving bowls. Top each serving with diced fresh tomato and chopped scallions.

FARRO AND KALE SOUP

$1\frac{1}{2}$ cups farro*

$\frac{1}{4}$ cup extra virgin olive oil

2 cloves garlic,
peeled and crushed

2 carrots, thinly sliced

1 onion, finely chopped

2 lbs. kale, stemmed
and chopped

1 15-ounce can
cannellini beans

1 $14\frac{1}{2}$-ounce can
diced tomatoes

1 Tbsp. basil, chopped

1 Tbsp. Italian flat parsley,
chopped

$\frac{1}{4}$ tsp. crushed red
pepper

$\frac{1}{4}$ cup Parmesan
cheese, grated

Bring a large pot of water to a rolling boil. Add the farro and cook on medium low heat until tender, about 20 minutes. Reserve 4 cups of the cooking water before draining the farro.

Add olive oil and garlic into large soup pot. Sauté the garlic until softened but not browned. Add the carrots and onion and cook, stirring frequently, until softened, about 7 minutes.

Stir in the kale and $\frac{1}{2}$ cup water. Cover the pot and cook approximately 10 minutes until the kale has wilted. Add cannellini beans, diced tomatoes, basil, parsley, and crushed red pepper.

---

*Farro is an ancient grain of Italy and can be found in most health food grocery stores and supermarkets.

Reduce the heat to low. Partially cover the pan with the lid and simmer for additional 10 minutes.

Add the drained farro and 3 cups of the reserved cooking water to kale soup mixture. Season with salt and pepper. Simmer for another 10 minutes over medium heat.

Ladle into individual bowls. Drizzle with extra virgin olive oil and sprinkle with Parmesan cheese.

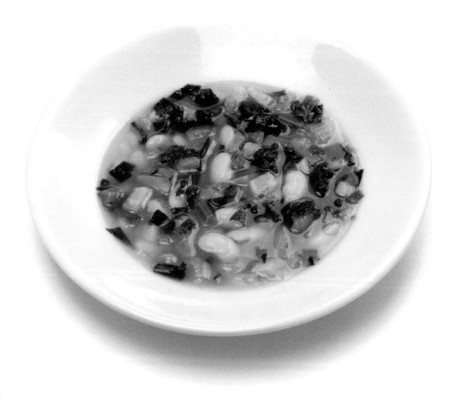

ITALIAN EGG DROP SOUP

Serves 2

4 cups organic chicken broth

1 large egg

2 cups organic baby spinach,
firmly packed and sliced

1 Tbsp. Parmesan cheese, grated

Place broth in a 2-quart saucepan and bring to a simmer.

In a medium bowl, whisk together the egg and Parmesan cheese.

Add the spinach to the simmered broth. Stir the egg mixture into the soup. Simmer for several minutes until egg is cooked.

Ladle the soup into individual bowls. Top with additional Parmesan cheese and black pepper to taste.

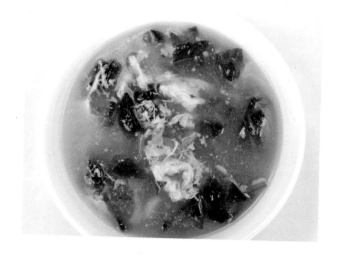

WHITE BEAN AND GREAT GREENS SOUP

Serves 4

1 Tbsp. olive oil

1 cup chopped onion

5 large garlic cloves, peeled and minced

1 cup escarole, firmly packed, chopped

1 cup spinach, firmly packed, chopped

1 cup Swiss chard, stems removed, firmly packed, chopped

5 cups organic vegetable or chicken broth

2 15-oz cans of cannellini beans, rinsed and drained

2 Tbsp. freshly grated Parmesan cheese

Heat oil in a large soup pot over medium low heat. Add onion and garlic and cook until tender. Be careful not to burn the garlic as it will have a bitter taste.

Add the greens and stir until slightly wilted, about 3 minutes. Add the broth and beans and bring to a boil.

Cover the pot. Reduce the heat to low and allow soup to simmer for approximately 20 minutes. Add more broth to desired thickness. Add salt and pepper to taste.

Ladle the soup into individual bowls and top with grated Parmesan cheese.

HEARTY RICE AND GREENS SOUP

Serves 6

1 Tbsp. olive oil

1 sweet onion, peeled and chopped

1 large stalk of celery, diced

3 large carrots, peeled and diced

4 cloves of garlic, finely chopped

1 cup of Wild, Whole Grain and Brown Rice Blend (Lundberg)

3 cups organic vegetable or chicken broth

3 cups water

3 cups kale, stemmed and chopped

1 cup Baby Bella mushrooms, quartered

1 15-oz can diced tomatoes, drained

1/2 cup Gruyère cheese, grated

Salt and pepper to taste

Heat oil in a large soup pot over medium low heat. Add onions, celery, and garlic and sauté until tender. Add rice, broth, and water and bring to a rapid boil.

Add kale; cover the pan and reduce heat to medium low and simmer for approximately 20 minutes until the kale is softened. Add mushrooms and tomatoes and continue to simmer another 20 minutes.

Ladle into individual soup bowls and top with cheese, if desired.

SIDE DISHES

KALE WITH CRANBERRIES AND ALMONDS

1 lb. kale, cut into $1/2$-inch wide strips

1 red onion, sliced

1 Tbsp. olive oil

1 pinch red pepper flakes

$1/4$ cup dried cranberries

$1/4$ cup toasted sliced almonds

Wash kale well in a sink full of cold water until any sand or soil has rinsed off. Change water and rinse again. Shake excess water from kale and dry on towel.

Heat oil in large skillet over medium heat. Sauté onion for 2 minutes, then start adding kale in small batches and stir until it all cooks down and you can cover the skillet. Leave cover on the pan and reduce to low heat. Steam until desired doneness. Stir in red pepper and cranberries and sprinkle with toasted sliced almonds. Salt and pepper to taste.

BOK CHOY WITH SHIITAKE MUSHROOMS

2 lbs. bok choy

1 Tbsp. peanut oil

1 Tbsp. sesame oil

3 green scallions, chopped bulbs
and some of the green

1 cup sliced fresh shitake mushrooms

2 garlic cloves, crushed

3 Tbsp. Tamari soy sauce
or Bragg's Aminos

Crushed red pepper, to taste

Cut off the base of the bok choy stalks and discard. Separate the remaining stalks and leaves. Chop the stalks into thin strips. Slice the leaves into 2-inch slices.

Heat the oil in a large skillet or saucepan over medium low heat. Stir in the onions, mushrooms, garlic, crushed red pepper. Cook, stirring often, until onions and garlic are translucent. Stir in the bok choy and sauce. Cook, stirring until the leaves are tender but stalks are still crunchy, approximately 3–6 minutes.

Bok choy can be served alone or over steamed brown rice if desired.

SAVORY SWISS CHARD

2 Tbsp. olive oil

2 cloves garlic, smashed

1 tsp. red pepper flakes

1 large bunch Swiss chard,
ribs removed and chopped,
leaves roughly chopped

Clean Swiss chard thoroughly. Remove ribs and chop into small pieces. Chop leaves into slightly larger pieces.

In a large sauté pan, add the oil with the garlic and red pepper flakes. Cook over medium heat until the garlic turns golden. (Be careful not to burn the garlic as it will have a bitter taste).

Add the chopped Swiss chard ribs and sauté until soft, about 4 minutes, then add the Swiss chard leaves and season with salt, to taste. Cook until the leaves are wilted.

Add a little lemon juice if desired.

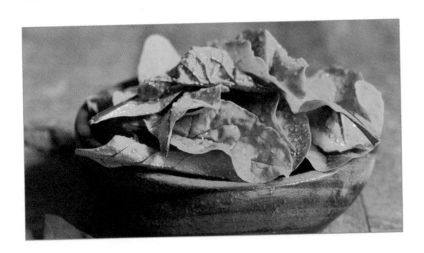

GARLICKY COLLARD GREENS

Serves 4

$2\frac{1}{2}$ lbs. collard greens,
stems and ribs removed

2 garlic cloves, minced

1 Tbsp. unsalted butter

1 Tbsp. olive oil

1 tsp. fresh lemon juice

Cut greens into 1-inch pieces.

Bring a large pan of water to a rapid boil. Add greens and cook for 15 minutes. Drain in a colander. Press out excess liquid with back of a wooden spoon. Set aside.

Heat butter and oil in a 12-inch heavy skillet over medium high heat until foam subsides. Stir in garlic and collards. Add salt and pepper to taste. Sauté the mixture, stirring often, until heated through, about 5 minutes.

Drizzle with lemon juice and toss well.

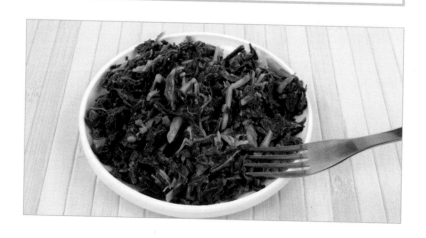

SPINACH, ORZO AND FETA

Serves 4–6

2 lbs. spinach leaves, chopped

3 cloves of garlic, minced

1 Tbsp. olive oil

8 oz. cooked orzo

4 oz. feta cheese, crumbled

1 Tbsp. fresh mint, chopped

Fill a medium sized saucepan half full with water. Add a teaspoon of sea salt and bring to a boil. Add orzo and cook according to package instructions, approximately 6–8 minutes, or to taste. Drain and set aside.

In a large frying pan, heat the oil on medium low heat and add garlic. Cook until the garlic is light brown, stirring often. Add the spinach leaves to pan and cover. Cook until wilted.

When spinach is wilted, add the cooked orzo to the pan and stir until well mixed. Add a bit more oil if necessary. Add crushed black pepper to taste. Add the feta cheese and heat through.

Serve immediately.

MAIN COURSES

HEALTHY ALFREDO SAUCE

Tbsp. olive oil

3 cloves garlic, minced

3 Tbsp. organic flour

1 cup organic chicken broth

1 cup milk (you can use 1% if desired)

$3/4$ cup Parmesan cheese,
freshly grated

$1/2$ tsp. salt

$1/4$ tsp. pepper

Heat olive oil in a medium saucepan over medium-high heat. Add garlic and cook one minute, stirring occasionally, until fragrant. Sprinkle flour into the pan and stir to combine. Sauté the mixture for one minute to cook the flour, stirring occasionally.

Slowly add chicken broth, whisking to combine until smooth. Whisk in milk, and bring the mixture to a simmer. Continue cooking until thickened, about 1 minute. Stir in Parmesan cheese, salt and pepper and stir until the cheese is melted.

Serve this sauce on Spaghetti Squash Casserole (p. 109) with a green salad of your choice and a loaf of organic grain bread to complement the entrée.

SPAGHETTI SQUASH CASSEROLE

Serves 4

2 large spaghetti squash

1 Tbsp. olive oil

2 cloves garlic, minced

1/4 cup scallions, chopped

2 medium size onions, finely chopped

5 large portabella mushroom caps, chopped

1 lb. bag fresh baby spinach

12 oz. organic mozzarella, shredded

Alfredo sauce*

Slice the squash in half lengthwise and scoop out the seeds. Place squash, cut side down, in a baking dish. Add 1/2-inch water and cover tightly with foil. Bake at 375° for 20–30 minutes or until easily pierced with a fork. Cool slightly. Remove squash from the skin using a fork and put squash into large bowl.

While squash is baking, heat olive oil in a medium saucepan over medium low heat. Add garlic, scallions, onions and sauté until tender. Add mushrooms and spinach and cook until spinach is wilted.

Add the ingredients from saucepan into the bowl with the squash. Pour Alfredo sauce and mix well. Pour half of the mixture into a baking dish and top with half of the mozzarella cheese. Add remaining mixture and top with remaining mozzarella. Bake at 350 degrees for 20 minutes.

*See the Healthy Alfredo Sauce recipe on page 108.

QUINOA STUFFED COLLARD GREENS

4 large collard green leaves

1/2 cup quinoa*

1 cup water

1/2 onion, diced

4 garlic cloves, minced

3 Tbsp. unsalted butter

2 Tbsp. olive oil

Salt and pepper to taste

1 Tbsp. red pepper flakes

1/4 cup fresh chopped parsley

1-15-oz. can of cannellini beans, rinsed & drained

1/2 cup Parmesan

Marinara sauce

Marinara Sauce:

2 28-oz. cans of crushed San Marzano tomatoes

1 onion, peeled and finely chopped

5 cloves of garlic, finely chopped

1 tsp. crushed red pepper

3 Tbsp. olive oil

1/2 cup fresh basil leaves, chopped

1/4 cup fresh oregano, chopped

1 cup water

Heat oil in large saucepan over medium low heat. Add onions and garlic and cook until tender but not browned. Stir in basil, oregano, and red pepper and sauté until basil has wilted. Add tomatoes and water and simmer over medium low heat for 30–40 minutes until thickened.

Bring quinoa and water to a boil. Reduce to a simmer, cover, and cook for 15 minutes. Remove from heat and allow the quinoa to rest for 5 minutes. Fluff with a fork, then set aside.

Bring a pot of salted water to a low boil. Immerse the collard greens, one at a time, until they are bright green and softened, approximately 20–30 seconds. Drain on paper towels. Repeat this step with all four collard greens.

Over medium heat, melt the butter and olive oil together. Add the onion, red pepper flakes, salt and pepper to taste. Cook the mixture until the onion is softened and translucent. Add the garlic and parsley to the onions. Cook for another 5 minutes.

Drain and rinse the cannellini beans. Mix gently into the onion mixture. Warm the beans, about 1 minute.

Put the mixture into a medium-sized mixing bowl and gently fold in the quinoa and Parmesan cheese until well combined.

Place one collard green at a time on a flat surface and add $1/4$ of the mixture to the center of the leaf. Fold in the sides, and then starting at the bottom, roll the leaf over the mixture until you get a rolled leaf that resembles an eggroll.

Repeat this step with each collard green.

Coat the bottom of the baking dish with olive oil. Place the stuffed collard greens into the dish, seam side down. Cover the rolls with marinara sauce, reserving some of the sauce to use prior to serving.

Cover with foil, and bake in a 375-degree oven for 25 minutes.

Remove the foil and bake for an additional 5 minutes.

Remove from oven and allow the dish to cool for 10 minutes. Top each stuffed collard green with a spoonful of the marinara and a sprinkle of Parmesan prior to serving.

---

*Quinoa produces its own natural deterrent to insects. Be sure to rinse it well before cooking. Some quinoa comes pre-rinsed, but I recommend rinsing it again prior to cooking to prevent stomach upset.

PASTA AND GREENS

Serves 4

1 bunch collard greens, stemmed and washed

2 Tbsp. extra virgin olive oil

1 medium red onion, sliced

$1/4$ tsp. red pepper flakes

2 garlic cloves, minced

Freshly ground pepper

8 oz. penne pasta (Use brown rice pasta for gluten-free option. Do not overcook)

$1/2$ cup cooking water from the pasta

1 to 2 ounces Parmesan, shaved

Salt to taste

Bring a large pot of water to a boil, salt generously and add the collard greens. Boil for 2 minutes. Using a slotted spoon, transfer to a bowl of cold water. Reserve water and set aside. Drain the greens and squeeze out excess water. Cut the greens crosswise into thin ribbons.

Heat the olive oil over medium heat in a large frying pan. Add the sliced onion and sauté, stirring often, until it is tender and translucent, about 5 minutes. Add a generous pinch of salt, the red pepper flakes, and the garlic. Cook, stirring, until the garlic is fragrant, about 1 minute. Add the collard greens. When the greens begin to sizzle, turn the heat to low, cover and simmer 5 minutes. Add $1/2$ cup water, cover and continue to simmer for another 5 to 10 minutes, stirring often, until the greens are tender. Add salt and pepper to taste.

Bring the reserved water back to a boil and add the pasta. Cook al dente, following the timing instructions on the package.

Before draining the pasta, ladle $1/2$ cup of the cooking water from the pot into the frying pan with the collard greens and onions. Drain the pasta and toss with the greens. Serve, topping each serving with shaved Parmesan to taste.

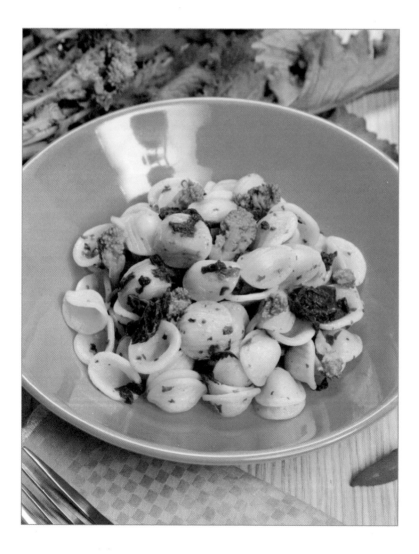

EGGPLANT AND ARUGULA
FLATBREAD

2 medium size eggplant, peeled and cut into $1/2$ inch cubes

2 Tbsp. extra virgin olive oil

1 tsp. freshly ground sea salt

$1/2$ tsp. freshly ground pepper

4 8-inch soft whole lavash

1 cup cherry tomatoes, halved

$1/2$ cup black olives, chopped

$1/2$ cup scallions, chopped

2 cloves garlic, minced

8 cups organic baby arugula

$3/4$ cup feta cheese

1 Tbsp. fresh lemon juice

Preheat oven to 450 degrees. Toss eggplant with 1 teaspoon salt in medium size bowl. Place salted eggplant between two paper towels and let sit for about 10 minutes. This allows the eggplant to release any bitter juices. Pat dry and return to bowl. Toss with 2 Tbsp. of olive oil, salt, and pepper.

Spread eggplant cubes onto a baking pan and roast for approximately 15 minutes until soft and browned. Remove from oven. Add the tomatoes, scallions, garlic, and eggplant into a bowl and mix well.

Brush lavash lightly with olive oil and place on rimmed baking sheets. Top the crusts with eggplant mixture. Sprinkle feta cheese over the flatbread and bake in preheated oven until cheese melts, about 5 minutes.

Toss arugula in a large bowl with 2 Tbsp. olive oil and 1 tsp. of fresh lemon juice.

Top each eggplant lavash flatbread with the arugula. Sprinkle with additional grated Parmesan cheese and crushed red pepper, if desired.

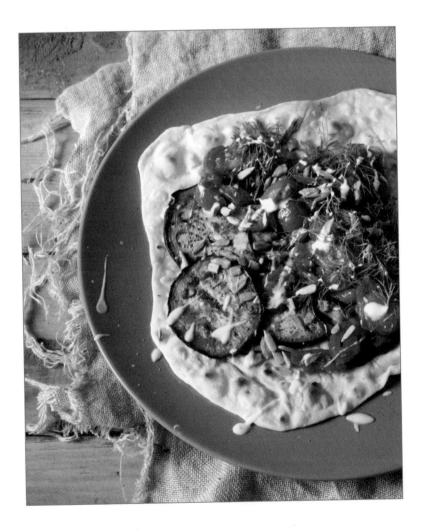

BUTTERNUT BEAN STEW

Serves 8

1 Tbsp. olive oil

1 large sweet onion, chopped

4 cloves garlic, minced

1 medium organic red bell pepper, chopped

1 medium organic yellow pepper, chopped

1 jalapeño pepper, seeded and minced

4 cups butternut squash, precooked and cubed

1 28 oz. can diced tomatoes

2 cups precooked black beans

2 tsp. ground cumin

2 tsp. ground turmeric

3 cups organic vegetable broth

1 lb. Swiss chard, stemmed and sliced thin

4 cups steamed brown rice

1/2 cup fresh cilantro, chopped

Salt and pepper, to taste

Heat olive oil in a soup pot on medium low heat. Add onion, red and yellow peppers, and garlic. Cook until onion is slightly browned and garlic is fragrant. Add the squash, tomatoes, beans, spices, and vegetable broth. Bring to a boil, reduce to simmers and simmer for 10 minutes with lid on the soup pot.

Separate the chard into three batches. Stir one batch at a time into the stew until wilted. Continue to simmer for 15 minutes or until the greens are tender.

Place 1/2 cup of cooked brown rice in individual bowls. Cover with stew and garnish with fresh cilantro.

If more heat is desired, add sriracha hot sauce to taste.

Resources

Chapter 2. The Good Ole Days When Food Was Food

National Institutes of Health

United States Department of Health and Services

Chapter 3. Organic Is the Best Choice

Renee Loux Prevention Magazine

www.prevention.com/food/healthy-eating-tips/top-reasons-choose-organic-foods

Chapter 4. Choose Your Produce Wisely

Environmental Working Group (EWG)

Andrew Weil, MD

Chapter 6. Set Your Goals

Carnegie Mellon University

Chapter 7. Stress Less

Harvard Women's Health Watch

Chapter 11. Here's to Juices and Smoothies

United Cancer Institute

FOOD DIARY

_____

_____

_____

_____

_____

_____

_____

_____

_____

_____

_____

_____

_____

_____

_____

_____

_____

_____

_____

FOOD DIARY

FOOD DIARY

FOOD DIARY

FOOD DIARY

Index

About the Author

Mary McAlary is an author, a realtor, a nutritionist, an organic health food specialist, a healer, a mother, and a grandmother. Mary is so many wonderful things to so many people because of one simple fact: She is a Fighter—An Everyday Fighter. Mary lives the ideology "pay it forward" every day and does so by sharing her story and sharing the knowledge she has learned on her path.

Mary McAlary was diagnosed with multiple sclerosis in 2004. She began traditional treatments, but her health continued to decline. In 2007, Mary sought out a holistic approach to battle her disease and her outcome has been remarkable. In 2008, she graduated from the Institute for Integrative Nutrition.

Mary believes that good health is attainable through organic nutrition and a healthy lifestyle. Today, her MS is benign, and she is feeling great. As a certified holistic coach, Mary enjoys sharing her knowledge for healthy living with others. Mary McAlary lives in Andover, Massachusetts. She loves spending time with her family, cooking, and expanding her knowledge of healthy foods and lifestyles.

Mary is also the co-author, with George Foreman III, of *The Fighting Spirit*, published in 2015 by Changing Lives Press.